allure
CONFESSIONS OF A BEAUTY EDITOR

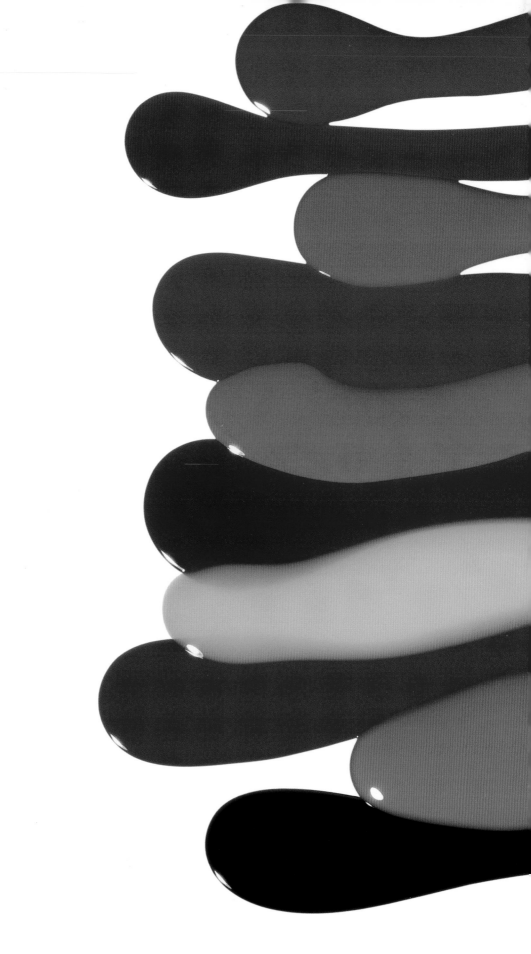

allure

CONFESSIONS OF A
BEAUTY EDITOR

Linda Wells

with the editors of *Allure*

BULFINCH PRESS

NEW YORK | BOSTON

Contents

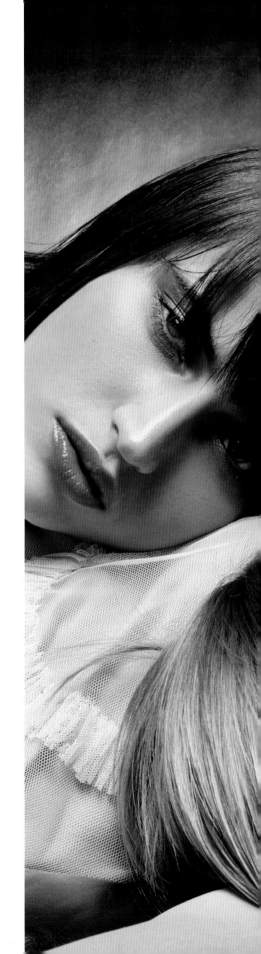

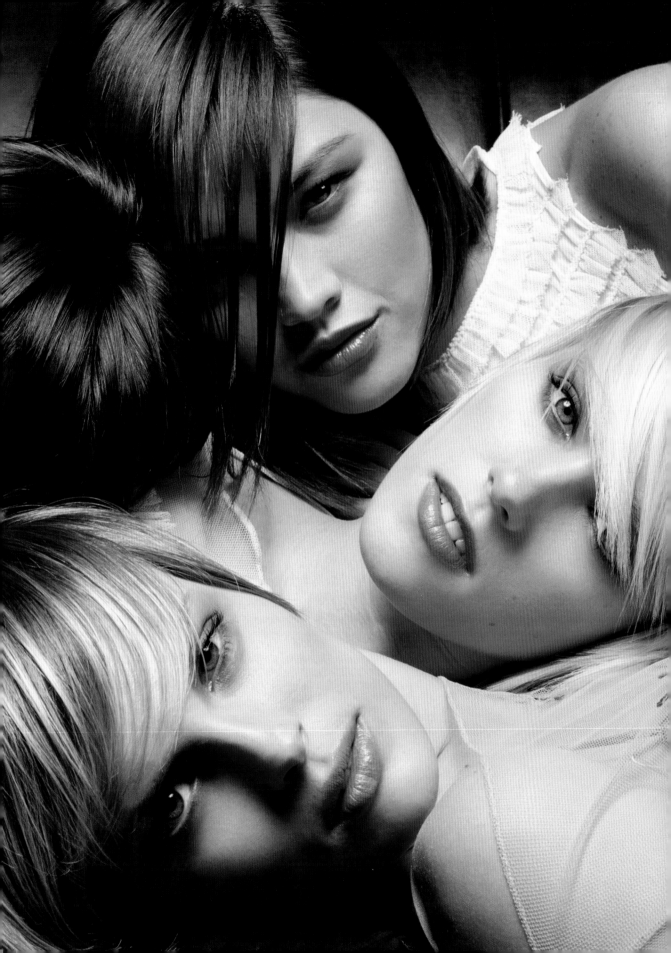

About three hours into my first day at a fashion magazine — testing lipsticks on the back of my hand, cataloging bottles of fragrance — I realized I'd found my true calling. Anyone who knew me before that moment would have laughed at such a thought; I was an unlikely candidate for beauty editor (well, beauty editor's assistant). At twenty-two, I came late to lip gloss, rarely did much more to my hair than wash and brush it, and had never once surrendered my nails to a professional. I admitted none of this to my skillfully made-up, perfectly manicured boss.

If I dig a little deeper, though, I see the early signs of beauty fascination. When I was about six years old, I spent three unrelenting months begging my parents for a vanity table with a frilly skirt that was advertised on television. I can still remember the jingle: "A little girl becomes a lady with a vanity all her own." Talk about a loaded message! At the time, I was in the habit of putting my hair up in sponge rollers before bedtime, learning to sleep through the lumpy discomfort. I dabbed on Tinkerbell cologne and wore dresses trimmed in lace. This phase was brief; by seven, I was back in pants, sneakers, and skateboard gear as if nothing had happened.

Later, I became preoccupied with skin, or — more precisely — zitless, blackhead-free skin. I spent much of my teenage allowance buying facial masks and electric brushes, eventually graduating to an appointment with a genuine dermatologist.

Beneath all this activity lay something more complicated than fastidiousness. I wanted to be clean and unblemished, yes, and feminine and grown-up, too. But more than that, I yearned to be pretty.

It's still a little embarrassing to admit that. The longing for beauty may be universal. If it isn't stamped on the X chromosome, then perhaps it seeds itself in the fertile soil of fairy tales, myths, and pop culture. Whatever the origin, many women eventually decide that the pursuit of beauty is either an impossible quest or a frivolous, shallow, even ignoble one. We stop pleading — out loud, at least — for the frilly vanity table.

And yet the desire lingers, doubles back, catches us by surprise. The fairy tales endure despite our best efforts to explain them away or rewrite their plots. Even those who possess great beauty are not immune. In an effort to comprehend their unbelievable luck, breathtaking models and actresses routinely tell stories about being awkward ugly ducklings.

The collision of longing and resistance is what makes beauty such a potent topic. When I started *Allure* in 1991, my mission was to demystify the subject and to make the tools of beauty accessible to every woman, regardless of the symmetry of her features, her age, or her body type. Back then the ruling queen was an Amazonian model with big hair, thick foundation, and heavy red lips: an intimidating ideal if there ever was one. Gradually, though, something called "the natural look" took hold. There was nothing truly natural about it if you added up the number of products needed to create the effect. But the impulse was refreshing: to enhance the face with colors that looked like they actually belonged there, to arrange the hair as if for a Herb Ritts photo shoot on the beach. The words "authentic," "easy," and "casual" became high praise. Perhaps most important, the aesthetic also began to embrace the country's racial and ethnic diversity as never before. Each year since 1991, the natural look has altered slightly, becoming more believable, more inclusive.

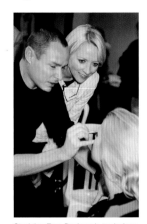

Studying Tom Pecheux's technique at Paris fashion shows

It has also become easier to achieve. In an earlier life, I was the food editor at the *New York Times Magazine,* where I learned to write recipes that noncooks could follow. I figured the same thing would work for beauty: If you can read and follow directions, you can be better looking. For me, the process of breaking down the big, messy desire to be pretty into small, manageable tasks makes it much less daunting and far easier to achieve.

Those tasks — or what we at *Allure* call tips, tricks, or, more seductively, secrets — are tempting because they are readily available and may have the power to transform. I'll try just about any new anti-aging cream, volumizer, or mascara if it seems better than its predecessor. Each one is a promise. I may not swallow every elaborate claim, but I do believe that some have the potential to make me look better, if only in the smallest increments. The bonus is that they often make me feel better, too.

The rituals of beauty, ultimately, can bolster a woman's confidence. Each morning when she peers into the bathroom mirror, a woman assesses her face and then applies concealer, blush, lip gloss, and mascara in an effort to emphasize what she likes and downplay what she doesn't. By making a woman feel more attractive, this simple routine gives her assurance, as well as a measure of control.

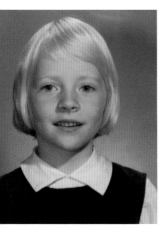
At six, this was the only haircut that made me cry

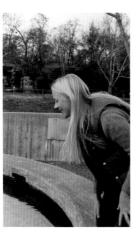
I had long hair and an L.L. Bean wardrobe at 16

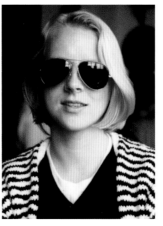
Wearing big aviators and a bob when I worked at *Vogue*

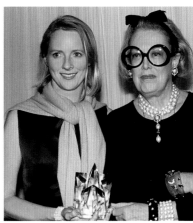
With Carrie Donovan, my boss at the *New York Times*

And yet so many women feel physically inadequate, focusing on perceived flaws in their appearance as their self-esteem drains away. I realize that no arsenal of tips, tricks, or even secrets can miraculously heal a wounded self-image. And I do not mean to minimize anyone's pain when I suggest the problem may partly be one of semantics. Words have tremendous power to shape our perceptions. The word "beauty" carries a world of insecurities about not measuring up. Beauty is often read as perfection: the 36-24-34 body, the flawless mane of thick, shiny hair, the Angelina Jolie lips — an impossible ideal. That's where "allure" comes in. Allure is something else entirely. It is a face with personality, a strong nose, or bright, mischievous eyes. It is a graceful gesture, a sexy walk, or a generous smile. Allure is unfettered by the conventions of taste and age. It is a bit of artifice pulled off with aplomb. Allure is an ephemeral element that comes from within and travels far beyond physical beauty. Yet it can be drawn out, cultivated, explored.

That's the best part. Because when fairy tales fail and perfect beauty is out of reach, allure is at your fingertips.

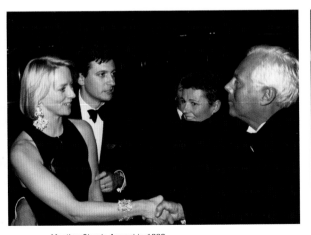
Meeting Giorgio Armani in 1992

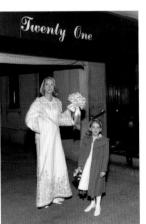
At my wedding in 1993

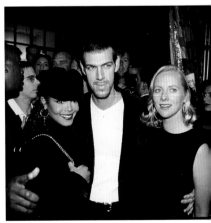
Seven months pregnant, with Janet Jackson and Kevyn Aucoin

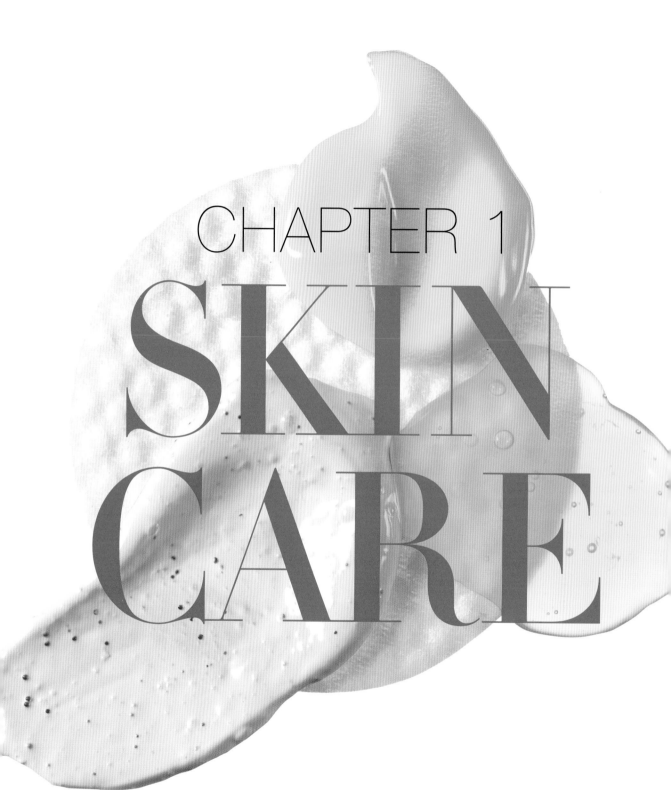

CHAPTER 1

SKIN CARE

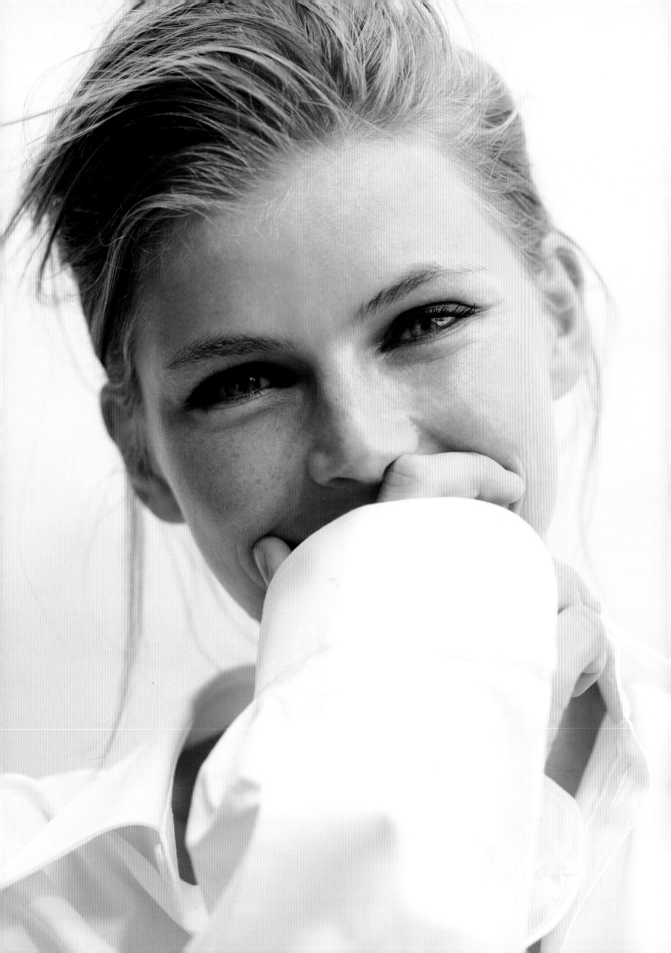

Every night before I go to bed, I open my medicine cabinet and gaze at the shelves, admiring the arrangement of bottles and tubes, lingering over each one. When I moved to a new apartment, one of the first things I set up was my medicine cabinet. Gone are the outdated prescriptions, the dried-up mascara, the six eye-pencil sharpeners, the detritus of thoughtless accumulation. The cabinet now holds only the perfumes and potions I love. The merely useful are banished to the cupboard below the sink, a jumble of cotton balls, nail-polish remover, and blow-dryer cords.

Medicine cabinets have always tempted me. I'll admit it: I have pried open the mirrored doors at other people's houses. But I'm not looking for dirty secrets; bottles of Vicodin and Viagra don't interest me. I want to know the clean secrets. Are they Dial-soap-and-Eucerin types, do they hoard little bottles of shampoo and conditioner from Marriotts and Hyatts, or are their shelves buckling under the weight of vitamin C serums, caviar creams, and Italian toothpastes? I fully expect guests to peer inside my cupboards, too. Whenever I have a dinner party, I make sure the cushions are fluffed, the candles are lit, and the medicine chest is ready for inspection.

When I was 11 years old, I'd sneak into my mother's bathroom and explore the shelves, pulling down the cardboard shaker of cleansing granules, the sandpaper-like hair-removal disks, and the blue paint-on, peel-off mask with the brush attached to the cap. I tried to figure out the mystery of growing up by testing the strange products of adult women — as if the answer were hidden in one of those jars.

On Saturdays, my parents would drive my brothers, sister, and me downtown. The boys, true to stereotype, tore into the sporting-goods store, my sister wandered the aisles of Woolworth's, and I'd plant myself at the pharmacy across the street, ready to spend my babysitting money on lemon-juice sprays and battery-powered face brushes. Fearing blackheads, horrified by acne, paralyzed at the possibility of body odor, I made sure my skin was clean and smelled of lemon wedges.

Now my medicine cabinet holds more moisturizers and wrinkle treatments than astringents and blemish ointments. Every night, I open the mirror door and stare, plucking the orange cleansing pad in the foil envelope from the top shelf, selecting the thick cream made from well-tended seaweed, choosing the serum that sweeps away imperceptible but entirely unnecessary cells from my skin. I climb into bed knowing that I've done what I can and go to sleep, letting nature and science do the rest.

Good-bye, cruel world (hello, sunscreen and antioxidants).

You know the old saying, "Prevention is the best cure"? We'd like to go back in time and shout it at our sunbathing 15-year-old selves through a bullhorn. Fortunately, there's plenty that can be done starting right now to make skin look its best — and prevent future wrinkles, sagging, and uneven tone.

IF YOU STOP READING at the end of this paragraph, it might still be worth the price of the book: Nothing will protect your skin more than the application of a broad-spectrum sunscreen of SPF 15 or higher (preferably 30). Every day. For the rest of your life. Be sure that your sunscreen or moisturizer contains zinc oxide, titanium dioxide, or Parsol 1789 — the broad-spectrum ingredients that block both UVA rays (the ones that reach deep into the skin to break down collagen and cause wrinkles) and UVB rays (those that cause actual sunburns and skin cancer).

YET ANOTHER REASON to take your vitamins: The other big culprit in aging is free radicals, which penetrate the skin to attack healthy cells. That's where antioxidants come in. The vitamins C and E, idebenone, and natural extracts including pomegranate, green tea, white tea, and grapeseed oil, now commonly found in moisturizers, all help protect the face from the main sources of free radicals — sun and pollution. There's also evidence that antioxidants can work from the inside out. One Australian study found that people who ate meals rich in leafy green vegetables had fewer wrinkles than those who had a high-fat diet.

THINK OF IT AS the Plastic Surgeon General's Warning: Cigarette smoking is hazardous to your face. If the specter of cancer and emphysema isn't enough to get you to quit, consider vanity — smoking unleashes a barrage of free radicals, and the constant puckering of lips around a cigarette produces fine lines around the mouth.

Trick of the Trade

Consider, for a moment, the Home Depot as a salvation for dry skin: According to dermatologists, a humidifier for the bedroom can keep your face from ever flaking off in the first place. They recommend machines that boil water into microbe-free steam.

Beauty Myth

The Myth: Drinking eight glasses of water a day will rehydrate your skin.

THE TRUTH: We also grew up reading this in our favorite magazines. Imagine our shock when we discovered that absolutely no studies have ever shown that drinking water makes skin moist. (That said, true dehydration does turn skin dull and peaked.) What does work: moisturizers that keep water from evaporating from the skin.

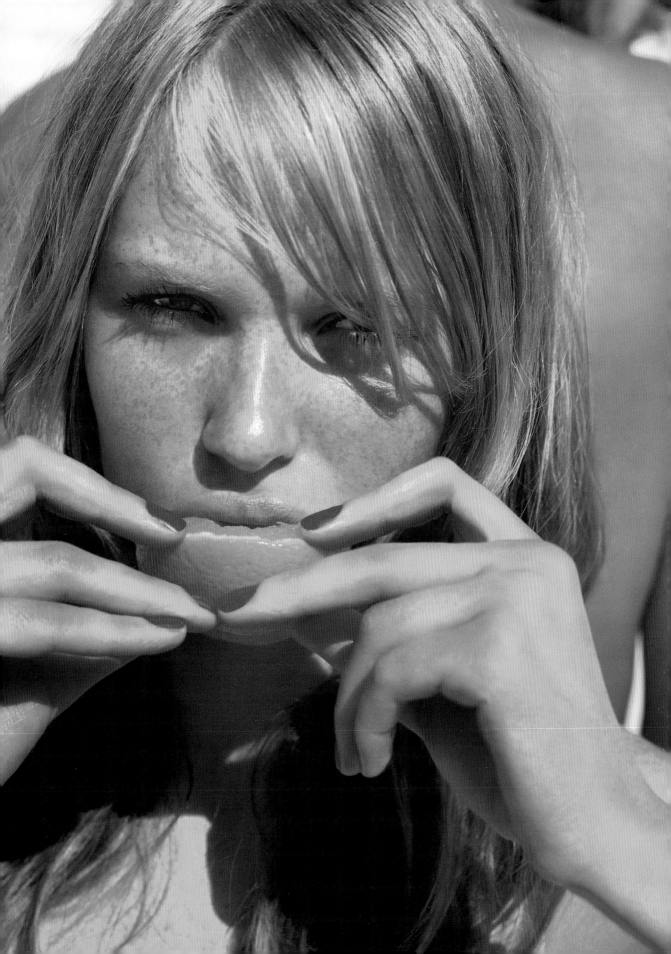

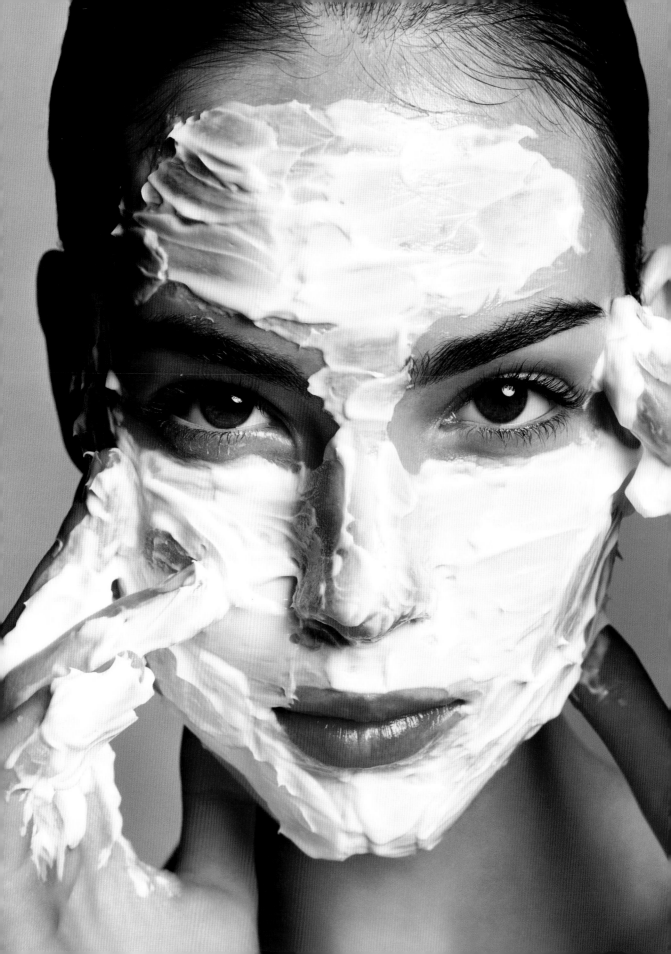

We've got washing our face down to a science.

A famous dermatologist once told us that the longer she was in the skin trade, the less she washed her face. It may run counter to our Puritan heritage, but the point of cleansing really isn't scrubbing or stripping until skin is raw.

THE ONLY IMPERATIVE is washing your face at night to remove grime and makeup. If you get an oily sheen overnight, by all means splash away in the morning — but twice a day should be the maximum.

DIFFERENT CLEANSERS suit different faces. Dermatologists love mild, creamy formulas because they don't irritate skin, but a foaming cleanser may be better for oily skin. And while it may seem as if cleansers don't sit on your face long enough to really do anything, ones containing glycolic or salicylic (also known as beta hydroxy) acid can provide a mild exfoliation that makes a small but meaningful contribution in the battle against fine lines.

WHEN LATHERING UP, be sure to cover lots of ground. It's easy to forget to work cleanser into the hairline, over the eyebrows, and down past the jawline, but those areas need attention, too. Always wash with lukewarm water. Hot water might feel good, but it can irritate skin and break capillaries. And forget about that "pore-closing" cold splash business. Despite the gospel according to your facialist, pores don't open and close.

SKIP THE TONER. When we say this in the magazine, we always get outraged letters from aestheticians saying skin isn't truly clean until it's been swabbed down. But dermatologists say

Cleansing 101

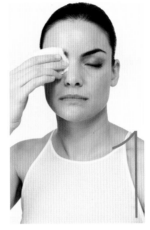

REMOVE MAKEUP

Apply a small amount of eye-makeup remover to a cotton pad. Gently wipe the pad across the lids and along the lashes, going over the area with a clean pad until it's makeup free (the only way to prevent black smudges on your towel). A little eye-makeup remover will blast away a lip stain or long-wearing lipstick as well.

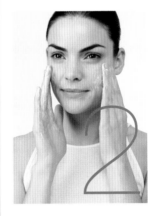

WASH FACE

Take a dime-size squirt of liquid cleanser, and rub it between your palms. (Most dermatologists recommend using clean hands instead of a washcloth, which, after several uses, could transfer bacteria to the face.) Massage cleanser into the skin, then rinse with lukewarm water.

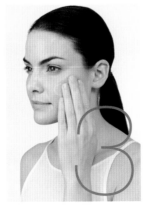

DRY AND MOISTURIZE

With a soft, clean towel, gently blot the face. Rubbing, dermatologists warn, can leave skin looking blotchy. Smooth a pea-size blob of moisturizer over damp skin on the face and neck to seal in water and conserve lotion — a tiny bit goes a long way on damp skin.

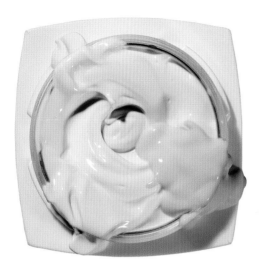

NOT EVERYONE NEEDS A THICK, heavy cream. You can tell if you've chosen the right formula by checking your face a few hours after trying it. If your skin looks shiny, switch to a lighter lotion or oil-free moisturizer; if it feels tight, first try increasing the amount you apply. If skin still feels dry, go for a thicker, richer blend that's more the consistency of butter than yogurt.

FIND A MOISTURIZER THAT DOES DOUBLE DUTY. Day formulas should contain a broad-spectrum SPF of at least 15, and after that, you can pick your weapon: antioxidants, anti-aging, anti-acne, you name it. Some dermatologist favorites include glycolic acid (which boosts cell

toner can be overly drying on all but the oiliest skin. If you can't resist the lure of the cotton ball, make sure your bottle is alcohol free.

There's a moisturizer for every complexion.

When staring at the shelves and shelves of skin-care products, it can seem as if there is a cream for every pore. But finding the right formula is actually pretty simple.

THE TWO BEST INGREDIENTS to look for are hyaluronic acid, a humectant that helps the individual cells stay plump with moisture, and petrolatum, which forms a barrier to keep water from escaping. For the driest skin, dermatologists recommend layering products with both.

Guilty as Charged

We slather on face creams like we're frosting a cupcake.

Yes, we've been known to coat our skin inch-thick with moisturizer. But a blob the size of a pea is enough to cover the entire face (add a second for the neck). The only exception: sunscreen. (For that, you'll need a teaspoon.)

Cheater's Guide

Too lazy to wash your face in the morning? Join the club. We gained a precious 90 seconds of sleep when top dermatologists assured us that our face doesn't really get dirty after lying in bed for eight hours. In the morning, rinse with warm water, pat dry, apply a cream containing antioxidants and a broad-spectrum sunscreen, and shock everyone by getting to work on time.

turnover), salicylic acid (to combat blemishes), vitamin C, E, or green tea (potent antioxidants), and soy (which battles uneven skin tone).

WHATEVER YOU CHOOSE, slather your moisturizer on immediately after washing your face, while skin is still damp, to seal that water right into place. There are only a few exceptions: If you are also using concentrated anti-aging or -acne treatments, apply those to skin when it's dry, and wait ten minutes before dotting on moisturizer to maximize penetration.

A QUICK NOTE ABOUT EYE CREAMS. We love to ooh and ahh over their pretty little jars and doll-size applicator spatulas, but the skin around the eyes doesn't require its own product. Regular moisturizer works just fine — as long as you are careful not to get it too close to the lashes. Anti-agers, however, do call for a separate eye formula, since many can irritate the area.

When it comes to anti-aging, our money's on retinoids.

We've tried every new anti-aging product from the rice fields of Japan to the labs of Long Island. But the creams that earn a permanent place in our medicine cabinet all have one thing in common: retinoids, the family of vitamin A derivatives including retinol, Retin-A, Renova, and Avage.

BESIDES FIGHTING ACNE and speeding cell turnover, retinoids are the one ingredient that has persuasively and consistently been found in clinical trials to spur the production of new collagen in the epidermis — and collagen is what keeps skin firm, smooth, and young looking.

Fly Right

The only thing worse than airplane lasagna is airplane air. The humidity level on a plane is lower than that in the desert (15 percent versus 35 percent, respectively). That's brutal to skin, but a few tricks can allow you to deplane looking rested, not ravaged.

1 After takeoff, spray or splash your face with water, and lock that in with a face cream and a lip balm. If you're sitting in a window seat, choose a cream with SPF 15 or higher — UV light penetrates glass, and it's intense at high altitudes. Reapply both hourly, or whenever your face feels dry.

2 If you're ambitious, the time in transit can be used for self-improvement. Makeup artist Bobbi Brown applies the thinnest possible layer of self-tanner to her face just before takeoff for a little extra glow at the arrival gate.

3 Forgo those salty pretzels, caffeinated beverages, and alcohol — they can exacerbate swelling in your legs and feet and make your skin puffy. Instead, keep your body well hydrated by drinking plenty of water.

4 A half hour before landing, remove any crud, germs, and who knows what with a facial wipe (followed by moisturizer). Curl lashes, and apply mascara, blush, and tinted lip balm. If you have a shred of self-respect, don't go near the fluorescent-lit horror that is the airplane bathroom.

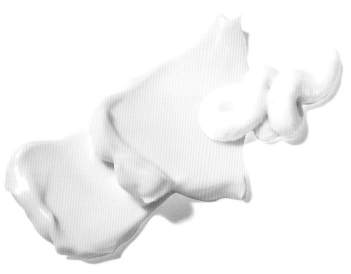

WOMEN WITH DRY SKIN and fine lines are usually prescribed Renova, which comes in a heavier, more moisturizing cream; oily skin may be better off with Retin-A Micro Gel. And retinol, the over-the-counter version of retinoids, is now available in concentrations (up to 1 percent) that approach the equivalent levels in mild prescription forms. (If your skin is extra sensitive, wait until skin is completely dry before applying a moisturizer that contains retinoids — a damp face may absorb too much too quickly for your delicate constitution.)

EVEN THOUGH THE WHOLE POINT of an anti-aging treatment is to generate collagen, beware of creams that boast collagen as an ingredient. It's such a large molecule that it can't possibly penetrate the epidermis and have any effect on the collagen in your skin. At best, it's a respectable moisturizer.

FIRMING CREAMS: There's no such thing as a face-lift in a bottle. Come to think of it, we've never seen a study suggesting there's anything close. For sagging skin, retinoids or copper peptides help boost collagen production and slow down aging — but unfortunately not enough to lift a set of droopy jowls.

How you wear it is as important as what you wear.

Once we found the right creams for our skin, we thought we were good to go. Bad call: It turns out there's a time (of day) and place (in the steps of your skin-care routine) for everything.

SINCE ALPHA HYDROXY ACIDS (also called glycolic or lactic acids) thin the protective outer layer of skin, they are best followed by a moisturizer with SPF 15 or higher during the day. And be careful not to overload — once a day is enough for AHAs.

BE CAREFUL LAYERING VITAMIN C serum with other acidic products: Vitamin C isn't pH-compatible with retinol, and both are ineffective when worn together. Plus, combining vitamin C with AHAs can be extremely irritating to skin.

RETINOIDS ARE THE VAMPIRES OF SKIN CARE: Not only does the sun render them less powerful, but according to dermatologists, they also make skin more sensitive to its rays, even days after you use them. Dab them on at night (followed by sunscreen during the day). Since redness is one of their side effects, lay off the scrubs and peels.

Beauty Myth

The Myth: Stroking creams upward will counteract sagging.

THE TRUTH: Gravity — the force responsible for holding the moon in the earth's orbit — is a tad more powerful than your fingertips. Skin will return to its original position the moment you stop pushing it around. (And no, if you make a face, it won't freeze that way, either.)

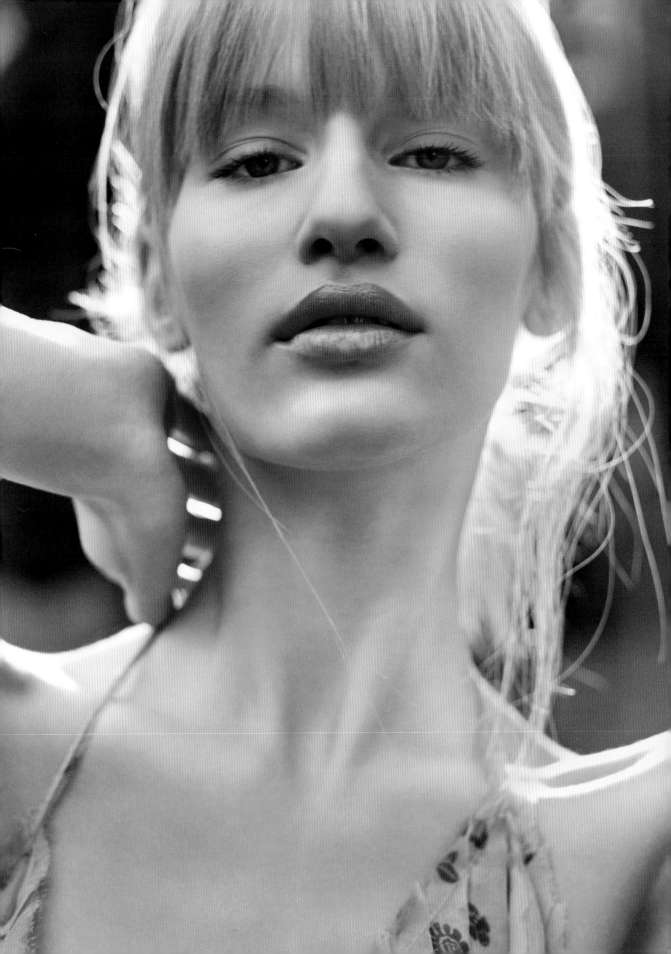

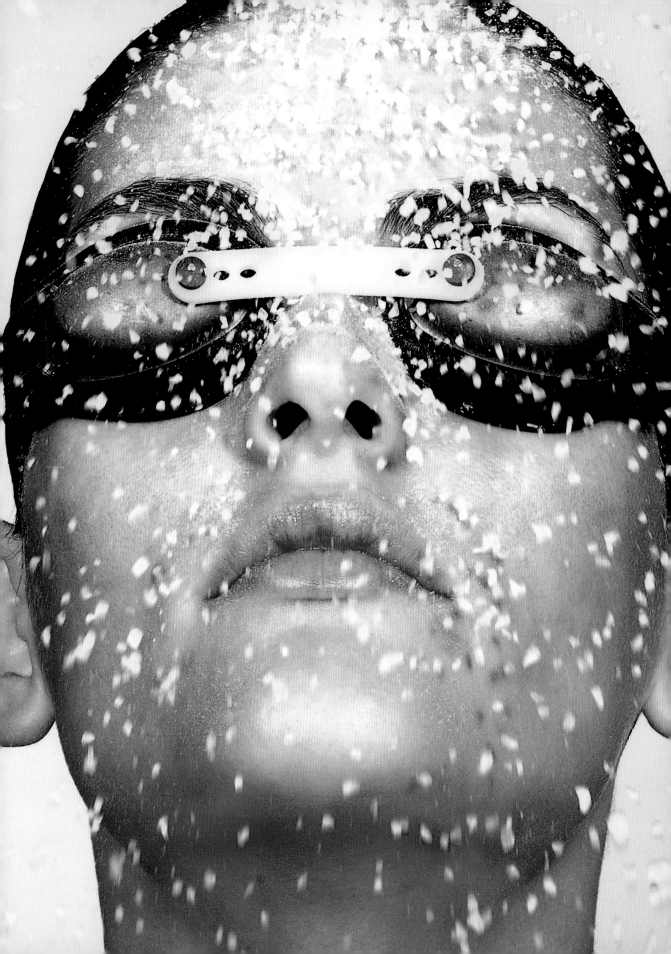

A little elbow grease goes a long way.

Exfoliation is the rare win-win scenario: It makes skin both healthier looking and more receptive to the active ingredients in skin-care products. The only losing proposition is grinding away at your face until it's red and irritated. You can put away the belt sander — there are gentle, effective ways to sweep away dead cells and leave skin glowing.

MANUAL EXFOLIANTS USE FRICTION to rub off the dull outer layer of skin. Few doctors recommend the trusty Buff Puffs of our youth anymore (too harsh, and they can harbor bacteria), preferring a once- or twice-a-week session with a scrub or paste containing gentle grains like sugar, oatmeal, or small synthetic beads. Skip the ground-up walnut shells or anything that feels sharp when rubbed on your palm — they are way too abrasive for the delicate skin on the face.

CHEMICAL EXFOLIANTS rely on acids (glycolic, salicylic, or lactic) to loosen those dead cells and sweep them away. The mildest versions come in daily cleansers. More intense formulas are usually scrubs or masks and should only be applied once or twice a week, depending on your skin's sensitivity.

Trick of the Trade

All good things must come to an end, and that includes jars of face cream. Most unopened bottles will stay potent for two years, assuming you store them in a cool, dry place. Opened ones will last no more than six months. Retinoid lotions, preservative-free creams, and antioxidant serums with vitamins C or E will start to lose their effectiveness earlier. And ingredients such as glycolic acid actually become more concentrated over time. If you detect a change in color or odor or feel a lot of stinging, toss the jar.

Anti-Aging Through the Ages

In Your 20s: Prevention

This is the time to start being vigilant about broad-spectrum sunscreen and antioxidants to prevent premature aging. While dermatologists don't usually recommend targeted anti-aging treatments at this time, women who've had a lot of sun exposure as children can consider an over-the-counter retinol cream at night.

In Your 30s: Exfoliation

In the 30s, the skin begins to thin — and become more vulnerable to the environment. In addition to sunscreen and antioxidants, this is the time to concentrate on cell turnover. Add a night cream containing retinoids or alpha hydroxy acids to your routine, and perform a glycolic peel or at-home microdermabrasion at least once a month.

In Your 40s: Stimulation

By this point, you probably see fine lines and the first signs of sagging. Dermatologists can offer stronger prescription retinoids (to increase cell turnover and stimulate new collagen), plus skin-lightening formulas (for brown spots). Home peels or microdermabrasion should now be performed on a weekly basis.

In Your 50s and Beyond: Firming

Sagging now joins wrinkles as one of the top skin complaints. There's no magic ingredient to lift lax skin (yet). But dermatologists recommend applying a copper peptide cream, which can help slow the fall, every night. You may also find that retinoids have become drying; a moisturizer with petrolatum or hyaluronic acid will help. Finally, consider a tête-à-tête with your dermatologist about in-office treatments. You may be ready to call in the big guns.

We love to play doctor.

After our second or third mild peel at the doctor's office, it was pretty clear that we don't need a medical degree to smear on glycolic acid, wait a few minutes, and then wipe it off. Cosmetics companies have figured this out, too, and have introduced a new generation of products designed to mimic certain in-office procedures.

MICRODERMABRASION: Dermatologists or facialists aim a pressurized jet of aluminum oxide crystals over the face to remove the uppermost layer of skin; at the same time, a vacuum sucks away the dead cells, producing a brighter, smoother complexion. The at-home version usually doesn't include any machinery (unless you consider your fingers little pistons), just a high concentration of crystals that are rubbed onto the face. While some experts argue that the vacuum is what stimulates blood vessels to produce new collagen, we're pretty impressed with the results of the home kits: After a month of biweekly scrubbing, our skin actually won us compliments.

GLYCOLIC PEELS: In what's sometimes called a "lunchtime peel," the doctor sweeps a solution of 30 to 70 percent glycolic acid onto the skin. Because the home versions rarely climb above 10 to 20 percent (to minimize the risk of burning), results aren't as dramatic or long lasting — but they can also be less irritating. The ones we like best leave skin pinkish for a few hours, then glowing for a few days.

WRINKLE TREATMENTS: Any company promising Botox in a bottle or collagen injections without a needle might as well go ahead and hawk snake oil. That said, some active ingredients can provide a little temporary plumping and freezing. The Argireline in creams trying to mimic Botox is supposed to inhibit the skin's production of an enzyme necessary for the muscle contractions that cause certain wrinkles; at best, they make skin feel tighter and discourage us from knitting our brow for a few hours. Wrinkle-filling creams contain tiny fibers that aim to spackle lines and diffuse light. They can make fine lines less visible, if only for a short time, but experts attribute this mostly to the moisturizers in the formula, which plump up skin.

Beauty 911

You changed your skin-care routine — and you've got the nasty red rash to prove it.

Temporarily shelve the new products, and switch to a creamy cleanser and a hypoallergenic moisturizer. Apply 1 percent hydrocortisone lotion on the area twice a day until the redness and irritation disappear completely. (Go ahead and call the dermatologist if it persists past the two-week mark.) If you haven't panicked and thrown out all the bottles, you can reintroduce the new products one at a time in two-week intervals to determine which one caused the reaction.

We pledge to give products a fighting chance.

If you want instant gratification, pick up a new tube of lipstick. Despite all those claims to erase years off the face in just days, skin products take time to produce results.

ACNE TREATMENTS may start to kick in after a few weeks, but resist the urge to lose patience and up the dosage. Too much salicylic acid, benzoyl peroxide, or retinoids can cause flaking and even more of the redness you were hoping to get rid of. If irritation occurs, switch to using the products every other night.

FOR ANTI-AGING POTIONS, it's reasonable to expect to see a softening of lines, especially around the eye area, after two months or so. (If more than six months go by and you don't see a thing, consider switching to a more potent regimen.) And here's a silver lining to a particularly dark cloud: The more damage you have, the more likely you will be to notice changes.

Beauty Myth

The Myth: Natural and herbal products are better for your skin.

THE TRUTH: Just as lots of substances in nature can be bad for you (like, say, poison ivy), most of the ingredients cooked up in a lab (such as salicylic acid and retinol) are highly recommended by dermatologists. They say the keyword to search for on a label isn't "natural," it's "noncomedogenic" — meaning the product is proven not to clog pores and cause blemishes.

Shopping for Steals

Fancy packaging and even fancier pricing rarely sway beauty editors, partly because companies frequently send us new products in generic laboratory containers. A few things to consider when deciding whether to scrimp or splurge:

How well do you know your face?

If your skin is particularly sensitive or unpredictable, it may be worthwhile to consult a doctor or a knowledgeable guide behind the counter. They also often hand out free samples you can try at home before you commit.

How much do you like to experiment?

Even a dermatologist can't say for sure whether salicylic acid or benzoyl peroxide is going to be better at eradicating those blemishes on your chin. At $4.99 a tube, you can bring home both and try each for a week.

How attached are you to certain ingredients?

Some, like botanicals, vitamin C, Parsol 1789, retinol, and certain moisturizers, simply cost far more than old standbys, like mineral oil and glycerin. If you love that hyaluronic acid makes your skin look as dewy as Gisele's in a greenhouse, keep in mind that it costs nearly a thousand times as much as glycerin.

How big a snob are you?

Dermatologists love the big-name-drugstore brands because they often work just as well as more expensive products — and usually print the results right on the packaging. But the derms don't have a professional opinion on how cute the bottles are; that's your call.

The 10 Commandments

1
Wash your face just enough to remove dirt and makeup, not to leave skin feeling tight.

2
You wouldn't leave the house without brushing your teeth — the same goes for wearing broad-spectrum SPF 15 (minimum).

3
You can use regular cream around the eyes; we often do.

4
Choose a moisturizer with antioxidants that protects skin from the elements.

5
Reapply moisturizer hourly when flying, if you don't want to look DOA.

6
Look for an anti-aging cream with retinoids. It works.

7
Apply anti-aging or -acne ingredients before any other products to keep from blocking their penetration.

8
More isn't always better: A pea-size amount of face cream is enough.

9
Exfoliate skin every week with a gentle scrub.

10
If you want real results, give products up to six months to work.

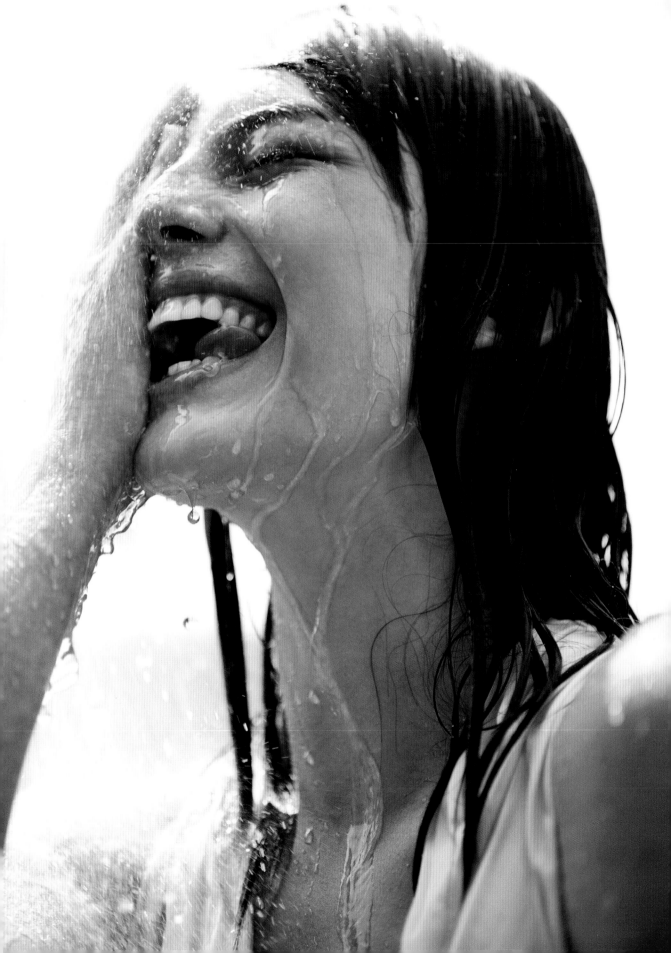

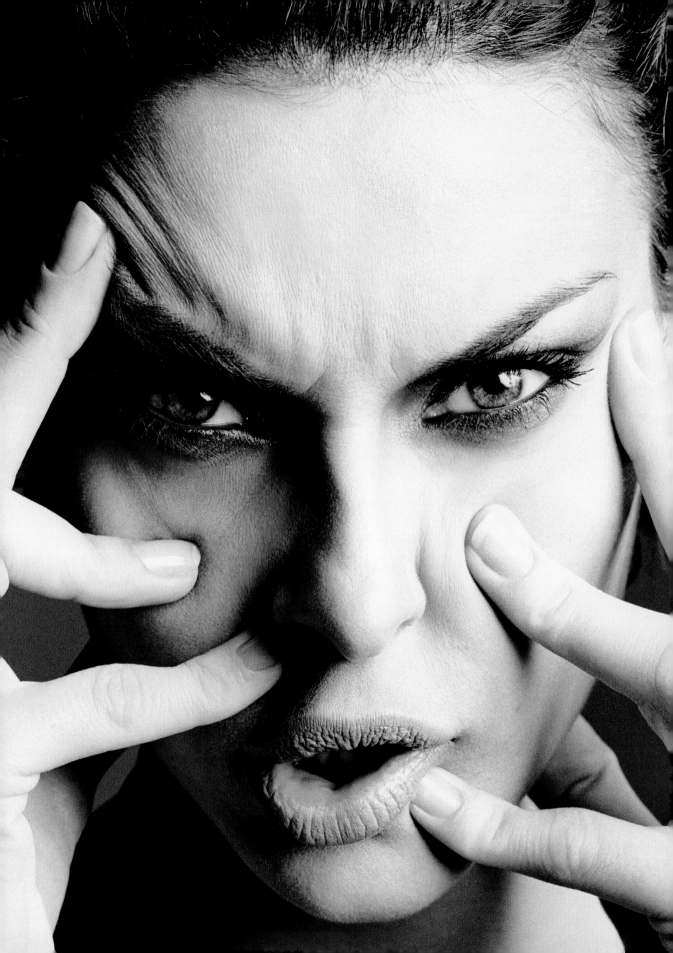

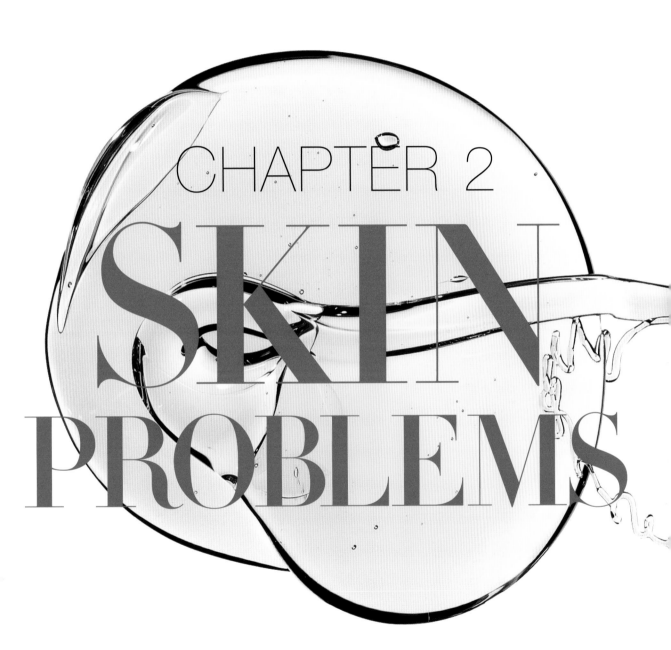

CHAPTER 2
SKIN
PROBLEMS

I ran into three people in the lobby of the Four Seasons Hotel recently who complained to me about their skin. Each had a similar story. "The magnifying mirror," said one woman. "I can't tear myself away from it. I just keep looking at my pores and poking at them until . . . this" — and she pointed to her blotchy chin.

One doctor has a name for the habit of scrubbing and probing the skin with Lady Macbeth vigor: "porexia." She's seen cases where patients become so preoccupied with their blackheads that they end up leaving scars. Those light-up magnifying mirrors certainly don't help matters. What is invisible at a reasonable distance is distorted up close. The face becomes a grotesque cluster of freckles, hairs, blemishes, lines, and crater-like pores, all ripe for dissection.

Those mirrors should carry warning signs like the ones on cars. Rather than "Objects are closer than they appear," the message should be something about flaws being smaller. Or maybe this: "4x magnification equals 4x humiliation." Hotels could even offer a few mirror-free rooms for those in danger of a midnight relapse in the bathroom with the sewing kit.

Still, those magnifying mirrors are enticing. They seem to offer a clear answer to the elusive question of what any of us really looks like. Is it the face in the candlelit restaurant or the one in the airplane bathroom (please, no)? The six-foot-tall wraith in the mirrors at Barneys or the thick, sallow creature in the doctor's office? It's no wonder that our myths and fables are furnished with mirrors that distort, deceive, and generally wreak havoc. By contrast, the magnifying mirror with its optic lens and cool white light seems clinical, objective. That's a comforting idea, but it's another trap. Those blown-up images bear about as much resemblance to the way anyone appears to others as a microscopic picture of the blood cells or an X ray of the molars does. They're all accurate, even scientific, but that doesn't make them complete.

Knowing the topography of your face with all its pores and human imperfections is not the same as knowing the truth about how you look. No mirror, however powerful, can tell you that.

Zits happen.

Monster zits still take us by surprise. God knows why, since studies have shown that more than 70 percent of women aged 25 to 49 had an acne attack in the past year — and that includes beauty editors who wake up to find an angry red bump between our eyes on the very morning we're supposed to accept an award from a dermatologists' organization.

THE FIRST, AND OFTEN BIGGEST, challenge is to resist the urge to scrub and scrub the blemish without mercy. According to Yale University dermatologist Lisa Donofrio, women past the age of 20 require gentler products than teenagers, and applying a treatment more than twice a day can break the skin, infect the surrounding area, and eventually form a crust. This in turn slows healing and increases the chance of leaving a red mark that lasts for weeks. Charming.

INSTEAD OF CAKING ON ZIT CREAM, start by washing your face twice daily with a cleanser containing up to 5 percent salicylic acid to unclog pores and reduce redness. Wait five minutes for skin to dry, then dab the pimple just once in the morning and once at night with a speck of a 2 percent salicylic acid or 7 to 10 percent benzoyl peroxide ointment (you can also try a topical antibacterial lotion or mask containing sulfur). This should kill the bacteria that caused the mess in the first place. And forswear retinols on the area for a few days; while they do help prevent blemishes, they also exacerbate the redness in an existing zit.

IF YOUR BREAKOUTS ARE BIG, UGLY, and prolonged and don't respond to traditional lotions, ask a dermatologist to pull out the big guns. For some women, that's a prescription antibiotic or sulfur lotion; for others, it may be oral antibiotics, the Pill, or in extreme cases, Accutane. Laser sessions, while expensive, have been proven quite effective in zapping away zits, scars, and redness.

WHATEVER YOU DO, remember not to poke, prod, or pop. Ever. Adult pimples tend to start far underground and almost never come to a head, so squeezing them will only make them bigger.

Trick of the Trade

To speed the healing of a pimple, crush an aspirin, and blend it with water to make a paste. Aspirin contains a high concentration of salicylic acid, the same beta hydroxy acid that's in countless blemish products. (Just be sure to dilute it with water to avoid irritation, and skip the trick altogether if you're allergic to aspirin.)

Beauty Myth

The Myth: Dabbing toothpaste on a zit can make it disappear.

THE TRUTH: Yes, toothpaste is drying — but it can also be irritating, and fluoride and tartar-control ingredients have actually been proven to make pimples worse.

Guilty as Charged

We've popped a pimple from time to time . . . and lived to tell.

Interviews with dozens, maybe hundreds, of the top dermatologists in the country have made it explicitly clear that popping pimples is a bad idea. But we don't always listen. At least we've learned that when we can't resist the urge to pop a pimple, there are ways to minimize the damage.

1 Examine the blemish. If it has a visible whitehead, you can proceed. If it's below the surface, abandon ship — you'll only force the contents deeper and make the situation worse.

2 Hold a warm, not hot, compress to the spot for five minutes to increase circulation and soften the plug.

3 Wrap your two poker fingers in clean tissues to keep from spreading bacteria.

4 Apply gentle pressure around the center of the blemish for a few seconds. If it doesn't burst right away, stop. Seriously.

5 If it does burst, disinfect the area with an antibacterial solution like benzoyl peroxide, which can also help dry it out. Applying salicylic acid to the area in the following days should finish things off.

BEAUTY SCHOOL
Facial 101

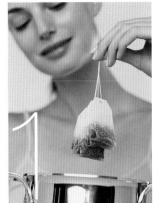

APPLY SCRUB

Pull hair back and off the face with a headband. Wash with your usual cleanser to remove dirt, oil, and makeup, rinsing the skin well and then lightly patting it dry. Drop four chamomile tea bags into a large saucepan of water, and while waiting for it to come to a boil, apply an exfoliating scrub with fruit enzymes like papaya. Do not rinse.

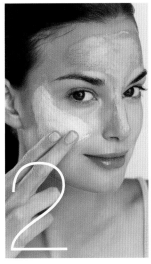

STEAM SKIN

Once the water is boiling, remove the pan from the heat. Hold your face more than one foot above it, close your eyes, and create a tent over your head with a towel. After three to five minutes, rinse off the exfoliant with warm (not hot) water, and gently blot the skin dry. Apply a face mask that's suited to your complexion —one with hyaluronic acid or glycerin for dry skin, sulfur for acne, clay for oily skin, or antioxidants for normal or combination.

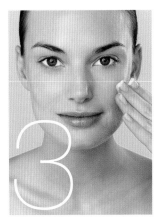

MOISTURIZE

Relax until the mask is ready to be removed (check the label for suggested time), then rinse it off thoroughly, and blot with a towel. While skin is still damp, rub on a thin layer of your everyday moisturizer — oil free for oily and combination skin, a richer formula for dry skin. If possible, wait six to eight hours before applying makeup.

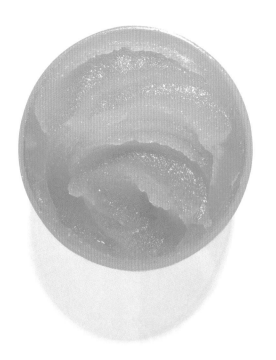

alcohol-based toner, which can irritate skin. Instead, try a drying lotion or mask with less than 5 percent benzoyl peroxide or sulfur a few times a week.

ON A DAILY BASIS, especially in the summer, the truly shiny may want to replace the moisturizer with a mattifying lotion. Ingredients like silica, clay, and various polymers actually trap and absorb sebum as it forms. Just be sure that the mattifier doesn't contain too much alcohol or witch hazel, which can overdry skin.

PURGE YOUR MEDICINE CABINET of hidden oils in foundation, blush, even pressed powder. If it doesn't say "oil free" on the package, it probably isn't.

A healthy glow is nice. A greasy shine? Not so much.

Perhaps the T-zone is really short for Twilight Zone: strange, unruly terrain characterized by maddening unpredictability. Here's a map.

DON'T STRIP AWAY THE OIL with an industrial-strength scrub — or your face will either rebel and shift into oil-producing overdrive, or dry up like an Arizona lawn in August. As with acne, it's actually better to bring down the attack. Wash just twice daily with a foaming cleanser, and resist the urge to swab with an

Trick of the Trade

Deep-conditioning treatments can be great for your hair — and not so great for your face. If you are prone to acne, be sure to keep hot oil or other heavy conditioners away from your bangs and hairline.

Beauty Myth

The Myth: You can shrink your pores with astringent or splashes of ice-cold water.

THE TRUTH: If only. Nothing has ever been proven to reduce them permanently, though remedies like clay masks and toners can make them appear smaller for a few hours. For the long run, dermatologists recommend retinol, salicylic acid, or alpha hydroxy acid to keep pores from getting clogged, forming blackheads, and generally looking more obvious.

We don't care if even supermodels get blackheads. We want ours gone.

The Chinese philosopher Sun-tzu's advice about knowing thy enemy also applies to blackheads. The first step in defeating them is understanding that they aren't simply a bit of dirt. The black is the oxidized product of oil, the equivalent of tarnished silver. No matter what you do, pores will continue to produce sebum — and will continue to be exposed to air.

START BY ELIMINATING FACTORS that can lead to clogged pores. Ditch foundations and heavy moisturizers that contain oil, which increase your chances of getting blackheads. Wash with a foaming cleanser (they're best at cutting through oil without being too harsh or leaving a film), then apply an acne medication over blackheads at night to unclog pores. The most effective contain 2 percent salicylic acid, which helps break down the adhesions between cells, softening existing plugs and preventing new ones. If you aren't getting the results you want, and your skin doesn't become irritated, step up to twice-a-day applications.

EXTRACTIONS, WHEN DONE PROPERLY, can indeed clear the skin . . . until pores replug in a few days or weeks. Dermatologists warn against frequent extractions, since all that prodding can cause pores to enlarge.

BEFORE CAMOUFLAGING BLACKHEADS or enlarged pores, fill them with something good, like a salicylic acid, retinol, or glycolic acid lotion. That way you won't develop little pools of makeup in your pores.

Get on Schedule

New Year's Eve. College reunion. Your ex-boyfriend's wedding. When you know you have a big event coming up, timing skin appointments is important.

Facials
Go one week before skin needs to look great to allow for recovery time from any postfacial breakouts.

Microdermabrasion
Have your first session three months ahead of the date. There's no downtime, but you'll need several sessions before you start seeing real, lasting results. Dermatologists recommend a minimum of four to six treatments spaced two weeks apart. And if you're just going to splurge once, go a day or two before the event for maximum glow factor.

Glycolic Peels
Go in fall or winter. While any redness usually lasts only a day or so, you need to stay out of the sun after a prescription-strength peel. Home peels with a lower concentration of acid can be done two days ahead of the event for the most radiant results.

Waxing
Schedule your session for one week before the big day—especially if waxing facial hair. You want to allow time for any redness or tiny bumps to subside.

Botox
Go two weeks ahead of time. It takes that long to see real results, and there can be mild bruising at the injection site, which needs time to heal.

We're all for being sensitive, just not on the outside.

More than 65 percent of women believe they have sensitive skin, according to dermatologist Patricia Wexler — but almost a quarter of those cases are actually caused by product overdose.

TRULY SENSITIVE SKIN has a very low tolerance for fragrances and preservatives, as well as anti-aging ingredients such as retinol, AHAs, vitamin C, and many botanicals. If this sounds like you, test any new product on a small section of your neck, then observe it for three to four days to see if a reaction occurs. As a general guideline, dermatologists advise sensitive patients to stick to products with fewer than 12 ingredients and zero fragrance.

LIMIT YOUR DAILY REGIMEN to a cleansing lotion, a moisturizer, and a PABA-free sunscreen (zinc oxide and Parsol 1789 are milder). Because they can be irritating, anti-aging or -acne products should be applied only one night a week; if the products still cause a reaction, try cutting them with an equal amount of moisturizer or over-the-counter cortisone cream. Those with sensitive skin should always wait at least five minutes after washing to apply anything other than basic moisturizer, as skin is more receptive to irritants when it's damp.

Dry is fine for wit and martinis, but not skin.

So, the moisture content of your face ranks somewhere between the Mojave Desert and a rice cake? If you nourish it with the right cream — and prep it with the perfect cleanser and exfoliator — your tight, itchy skin can be turned around within a week or so.

ALWAYS USE A CREAMY CLEANSER on the face, and follow with a cool water rinse. (Hot water strips moisture from the skin.) Then, while your skin is still damp, rub in a thick moisturizer containing petrolatum or glycerin — barriers that hold water in the skin. If that's not enough, layer a lightweight gel containing hyaluronic acid underneath. And in the evenings, smooth a cream containing exfoliating urea over extra-dry patches.

LAYERS OF DEAD CELLS — common to dry skin — can plug up pores, blocking the absorption of moisture from creams. Exfoliate weekly with a gentle scrub.

DRYING INGREDIENTS, such as clay and alcohol, only make the sting of flaking, water-deprived skin worse. Avoid them with the same zeal you would a bad blind date.

Cheater's Guide

Since the neck-and-shoulder-massage part of facials only lasts five minutes, and the rest tends to make us break out, we aren't all that inclined to schedule them before major events. Dermatologist Leslie Baumann taught us another way to get skin glowing — one that isn't for the faint of heart (or the sensitive of skin). One week before the big day, ask your dermatologist for permission to cake on a thick layer of Retin-A two or three nights in a row. You may look like a snake molting for the next couple of days, but skin will look bright and new in time for your moment.

Combination skin: The one legitimate excuse for buying twice as many products.

Many dermatologists consider combination skin to be a triumph of marketing — and not very meaningful from a biological standpoint. For women who consider it plenty meaningful when gazing into the mirror at a greasy forehead and parched cheeks, there is a simple solution: Follow the rules for oily skin on the T-zone and for dry skin everywhere else. After washing with a foaming cleanser, slick moisturizer only on the cheeks and around the eyes (or choose an oil-free formula for the whole face, then follow with a thicker cream where needed). Just be sure that all of the ingredients for oily skin — benzoyl peroxide, salicylic acid, sulfur, and clay — don't touch the dry parts.

TOP FIVE REASONS
To See a Dermotologist

1. That mole on your shoulder seems to be growing.

Yearly checkups are crucial to catch skin-cancer lesions, which may hide on the lower back, on the scalp, or even between the toes or may masquerade as a patch of dry skin. When detected early, the disease has a one-in-five cure rate.

2. You want that pimple gone — now.

When patience is not an option, a dermatologist can inject the pimple with cortisone, a steroid that stops the swelling and reduces redness immediately. A cystic pimple that would have taken two to three weeks to disappear on its own will be at least 50 percent better within hours of the shot and almost entirely gone the next day. Plus, you're less likely to scar or develop a dark mark than if you had let the blemish run its course.

3. Your skin flushes and stays that way.

Red wine makes it worse; so do spicy foods, vigorous exercise, and hot showers. For the 14 million Americans who suffer from rosacea, only a dermatologist can offer relief. The condition is fairly difficult to diagnose without a professional, since its chronic facial flushing and small red bumps mimic sensitive skin or acne. No cure exists, but a combination of antibiotics, prescription creams, and lasers can dramatically minimize the symptoms.

4. Your skin has done a 180 from oily to dry (or vice versa).

Sometimes skin plays against type: Dry skin erupts in zits, oily skin becomes flaky, normal skin acts sensitive. Most women notice changes as they move through their 20s, and by their 30s they often experience renewed breakouts (because of pregnancy or certain birth control pills). A dermatologist can help you determine the cause and suggest a treatment.

5. The spider veins in your legs have turned into a web.

Sarongs and self-tanner might conceal a tangle of tiny veins, but only a doctor can banish them for good. Sclerotherapy, also known as saline or detergent injections, dissolves both tiny veins and thick, ropy varicose ones. It takes three or four treatments and may need to be repeated after several years, but it's still the gold standard. While dermatologists can zap some veins with lasers, the ones in the legs may run too deep or be too large for lasers to penetrate; however, facial veins — which tend to be thinner and closer to the surface — are perfect candidates for the treatment.

A half gallon of foundation isn't the only way to get perfectly even skin.

There are about as many causes of red skin as there are rumors in Hollywood. These tricks will spare you the flush of embarrassment.

IF HIGH-POWERED ANTI-AGING CREAMS like retinol and glycolic acid are at fault, you can dilute them with regular moisturizer or cut back application to every other night. If that doesn't do it, you may want to consider switching active ingredients — soy, kinetin, and grape-seed extract are both effective and gentle.

ANOTHER CAUSE OF BLOTCHINESS is the inflammation of tiny blood vessels in the face. Unlike larger, more prominent broken capillaries, they're actually just dilated — usually because of too much sun, caffeine, alcohol, or cigarettes. Ask your doctor for a prescription anti-inflammatory. For stubborn cases, both Intense Pulsed Light and lasers can vaporize the contents of the vessels, causing them to collapse and dissolve.

IF YOUR FLUSH CAME FROM WAXING or a chemical peel, a 1 percent hydrocortisone cream can reduce redness (just don't apply to broken skin).

ROSACEA SUFFERERS NEED to avoid vasodilators — spicy foods, alcohol, aspirin, and the sun — which trigger blood vessels to expand. If over-the-counter solutions leave you seeing red, see a dermatologist.

AND FINALLY, you may have your parents to thank for that red face of yours. Do yourself a favor: Instead of therapy sessions, get thee to a dermatologist, who can cure at least *one* of your scars from childhood.

Dark circles and undereye bags may be hard to look at, but they're easy to hide.

We have a few key strategies for mornings when we have to look bright eyed (bushy tails are so over).

IF ONLY DARK CIRCLES could be wiped away with makeup remover like so much migrating mascara. Unfortunately, DNA is a bit more stubborn — and yes, a predisposition to broken blood vessels or hyperpigmentation are two more things you can blame on

Beauty 911

After waxing, all the hair above your lip is gone — and so is the top layer of skin.

If your upper lip is pink and swollen, start by applying a cold compress to the area for five minutes to soothe the skin. Then layer on 1 percent hydrocortisone cream morning and night until the irritation subsides, usually in less than a week. (If the skin is raw, hold off on the hydrocortisone for a few days, and apply antibiotic ointment instead.) Don't apply makeup or concealer to the area until the redness is gone; it might make the inflammation worse. And remember in the future to forswear waxing if you're using a prescription retinoid or Accutane.

your parents. While creams haven't shown much effect in reducing the bruised look, there are three prime ingredients to look for if you want a fighting chance: retinol (which thickens skin, making it harder to see underlying darkness), hydroquinone (which lightens the pigment over time), and vitamin K (which helps reduce broken blood vessels).

LACK OF SLEEP RAISES cortisol levels — which causes skin to retain fluid, among other unpleasantness. Drink a big glass of water before you hit the sack at 2 A.M.; it will reduce puffiness by decreasing the amount of salt in the body. Then sleep on a thick pillow to elevate the head and keep fluid from settling under the eyes. In the morning, if your counterattack hasn't worked, steep tea bags in hot water, chill in the fridge, and then rest them on the eye area — the tannins in black tea help reduce bloat. And before heading out to work bleary eyed, dab on an eye cream that contains both caffeine (to combat swelling) and light-diffusing particles (to distract your boss from the fact that you partied half the night).

If only the hair on our heads grew as quickly as the pesky ones above our lips.

In the past few years, Brazilian bikini waxes have become a socially acceptable topic of conversation — yet you'll rarely find us discussing the removal of rogue whiskers. The time has come to blow the cover on one of the more embarrassing beauty realities: the mustache and the billy goat beard.

UNDER NO CIRCUMSTANCE should a razor go anywhere near your face, not even in the case of a dating emergency. Stubble is bad enough on your shins.

DEPILATORY CREAMS ARE FAST AND CHEAP — and stink to high heaven. Rosin, the active ingredient, can cause irritation, so be sure to test a small area behind your ear first. (Sound like a pain? Consider that a reaction usually lasts three to four days — you'll agree it's better to have a red stripe hidden by your hair than slashed across your face.) Results last somewhere between one and three weeks, depending on how fast your hair grows.

WAXING LEAVES SKIN FUZZ FREE for up to a month, but it does turn skin pink and slightly bumpy for several hours (end-of-the-day appointments are key). The bad news is that, unlike the hair on your legs, facial hair won't grow in finer or blonder after waxing; but at least it won't become any coarser. Just be sure to gently exfoliate the area every other day to prevent ingrowns.

TWEEZING A FEW STRAYS NEVER HURT ANYONE, as long as the hairs are meticulously yanked out by the root — not broken off somewhere in between, which makes ingrowns more likely. The tweezer of choice is a slant-head model, and the best time to do it is right after a shower, when the hair slips out more easily.

THE LIP AND CHIN ARE FAST becoming one of the most popular places on the body for laser hair removal and electrolysis (to find an experienced electrolysist, ask your dermatologist). Because the area is so tiny, it isn't as expensive as tackling, say, an entire leg, and results from one session (for electrolysis) to four to six sessions (for laser) can be pretty close to permanent.

The 10 Commandments

1
Treat a zit with twice-daily doses of salicylic acid or benzoyl peroxide. Do not pick.

2
There is no miracle cure for blackheads, just preventive measures to keep pores from clogging in the first place.

3
Gentle exfoliation helps dry skin hold on to moisture.

4
Eradicate shine with drying lotions and masks.

5
The fewer ingredients in a product, the better it is for sensitive skin.

6
To treat blotchiness, avoid hot showers, alcohol, and spicy foods.

7
Eye bags can be banished. Dark circles can't — that's what concealer is for.

8

Tackle facials, peels, and microdermabrasion at least a week before a big event to allow for any irritation to disappear.

9
No matter how big the mustache, never raise a razor to your face.

10
Some problems are too big for skin-care products. Know when to go to the dermatologist.

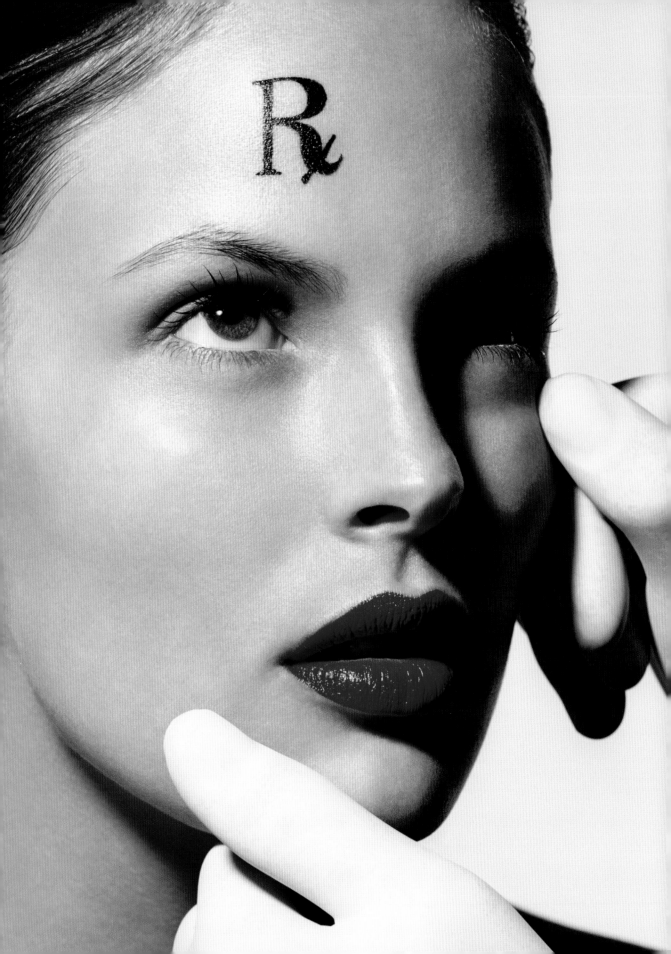

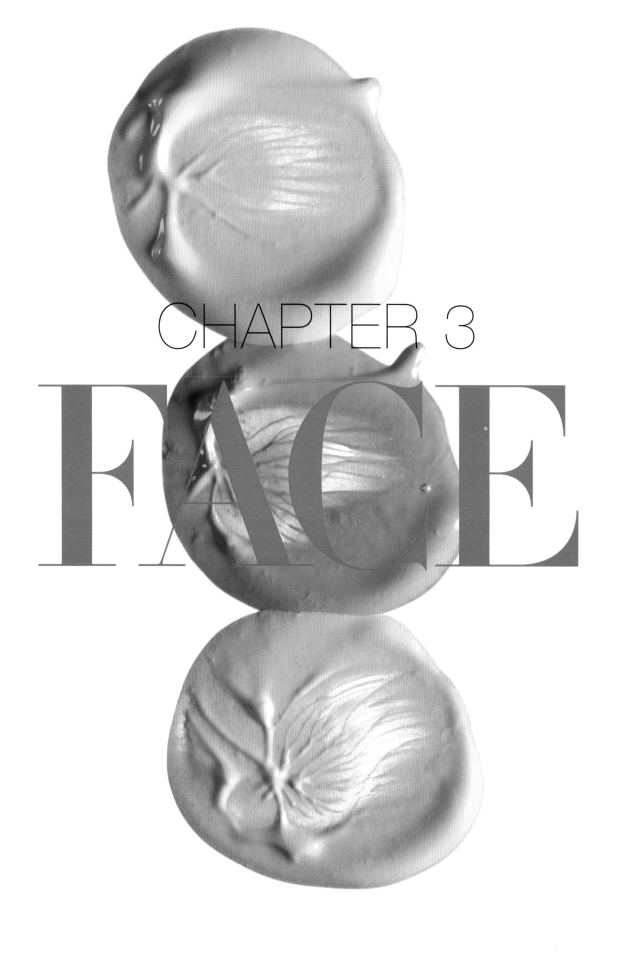

CHAPTER 3

FACE

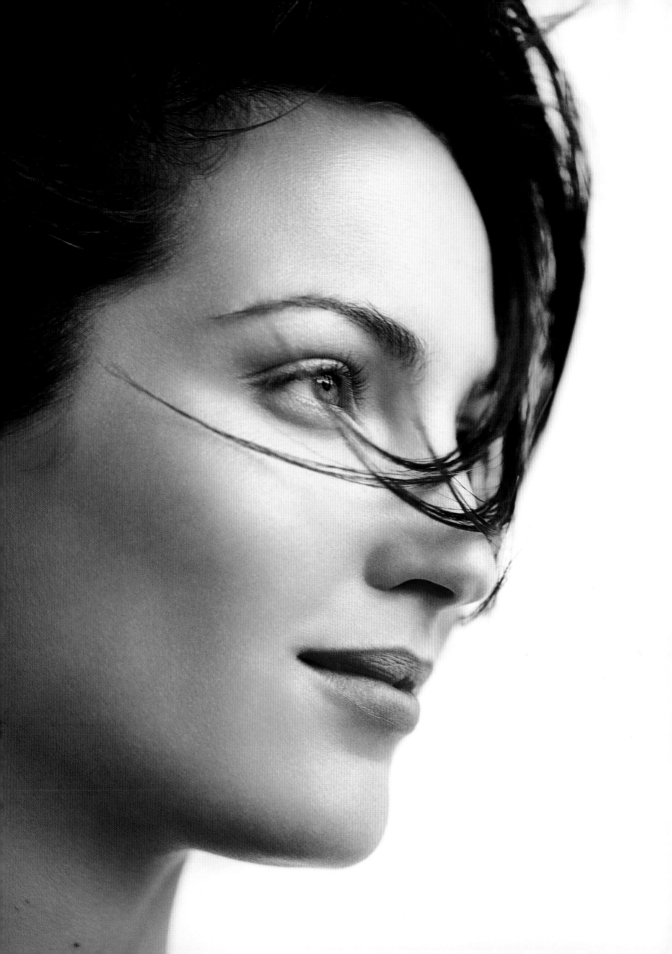

Everything that scares me about makeup could be summed up in one word: foundation. It is artificial, crude, heavy, and altogether unappealing. No wonder people call it base. I can still remember the way the sponge in my grandmother's compact of pancake makeup smelled, a sick musty odor with a touch of rose perfume. I loved my grandmother, and perhaps this memory should conjure up some sweet sense of nostalgia, but it doesn't. The makeup sponge was fleshy and lurid and not at all like her. Even the way people talk about foundation — "creating a smooth canvas," "building a base," and the wretched "applying pancake" — sounds antiquated.

Needless to say, I never touched the stuff. Instead, I'd just pat concealer on my undereye circles and hope for the best. Whenever I had to submit my face to a professional makeup demonstration for work, I'd plot my escape to the nearest bathroom (seventh floor of Bergdorf's, second floor of Bloomingdale's, and, for desperate cases that required a private sink, the lobby of the Waldorf-Astoria).

As if answering my prayers, some of the top makeup artists decided to dispense with foundation about a decade ago, declaring it fake and mask-like. They replaced it with concealer, which they'd smear on the model's blemishes, scars, and freckles, explaining how women had to break the habit of plastering their face (and neck and chest and . . . where does it stop?) with base.

Makeup artists didn't have to fret much over the demise of foundation. After all, they worked on eighteen-year-old models who had little or nothing to hide. What concealer couldn't cover, computer retouching would, down to the models' tiniest flaws. How nice for them.

Those foundation-free years may not have been as kind to the rest of us, but they did bring about some major changes in makeup. A new kind of foundation has emerged that is base no more. It's sheer, easy to wear, and bears cozier names, such as "Gentle Light Makeup," "Ultra-Comfort Skin-Illuminating Makeup," or simply "tinted moisturizer." The best label I've seen on a bottle yet is "Non-fiction," and it's just what we need: makeup that seems factual and clear. Even makeup artists and models are dipping into these creamy, realistic-looking products. Now I can use foundation without an escape plan.

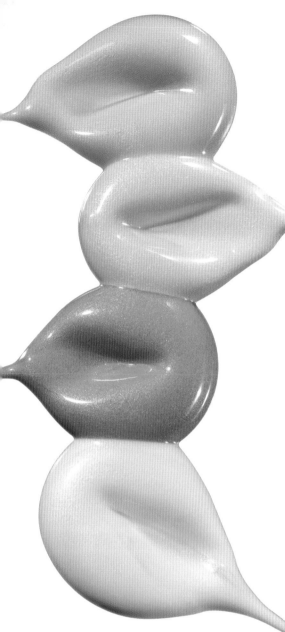

The "natural look" can require a lot of makeup.

When we hear someone say for the thousandth time how ironic it is that beauty editors don't wear makeup, we just smile and nod. The truth is that we've just picked up enough tricks over the years so that the foundation, concealer, blush, highlighter, and powder look like just a little glow.

EXFOLIATE, EXFOLIATE, EXFOLIATE. Even the best makeup in the world will look like dirt if it's applied on top of skin that is dry, dull, or flaky. Regular sloughing, whether with chemicals (like glycolic acid home peels or nightly application of retinoids) or a gentle, grainy scrub, will make skin more naturally radiant — and allow you to wear less makeup.

SOME MAKEUP ARTISTS BELIEVE IT'S HERESY to apply foundation directly to bare skin. They say makeup primer creates a remarkably smooth surface. If you don't want to add an extra step and a new product, just massage moisturizer onto clean skin. Makeup will then seem to melt into the face rather than sit awkwardly on top of it.

THE FAMOUS RULE ABOUT GETTING READY, then removing one accessory before you leave the house applies just as well to makeup. After you've done your face, turn away from the mirror, then quickly turn back. You might be surprised to see that your blush suddenly looks too bright, or the shimmer on your eyes is more disco than dazzling. A light dusting of powder will tone it down.

Beauty Myth

The Myth: You should always test foundation on the back of your hand.

THE TRUTH: Because your hands have been exposed to more UV light and a lot less exfoliation, they are usually darker than your face. It's best to draw stripes of foundation on the jawline, then examine them in natural light.

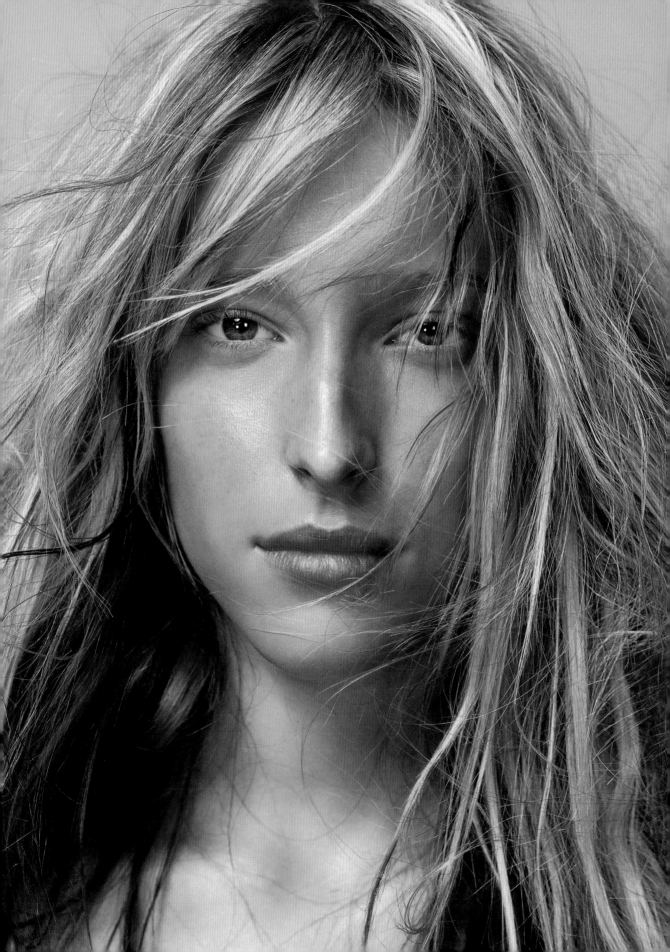

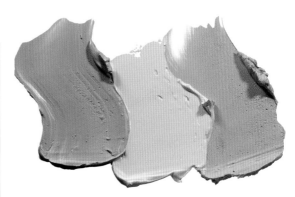

BEAUTY SCHOOL

Flawless Skin 101

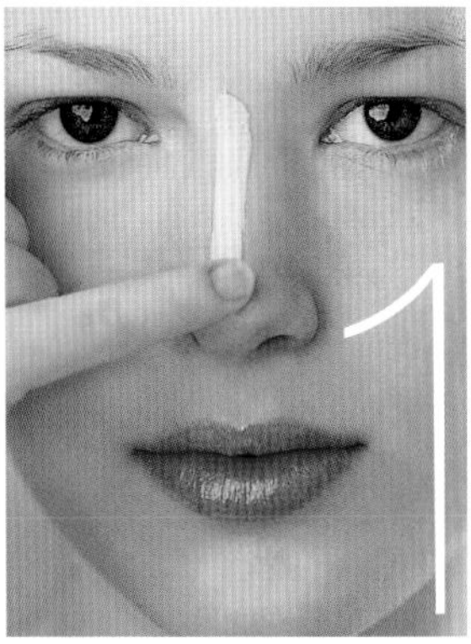

DAB IT ON

Start with a perfectly clean, freshly moisturized face. Pour a dime-size amount of foundation into the palm to warm it up. Then dot it onto blemishes and any place that's darker or redder than the rest of the face — usually on the chin, under the eyes, on and around the nose, and at the corners of the mouth.

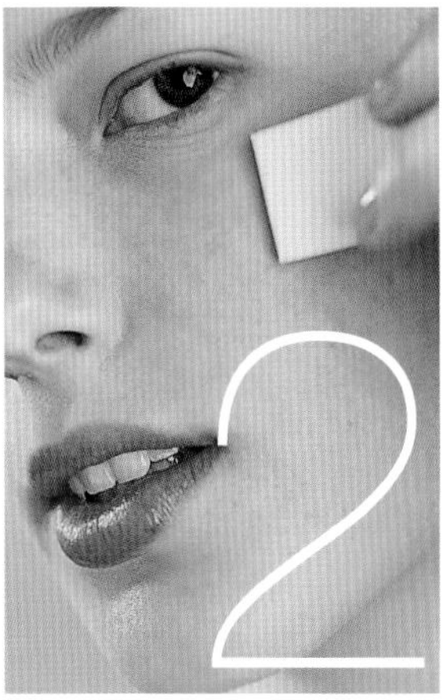

RUB IT IN

Begin in the middle of the face, and move outward, smoothing foundation with fingers, a nylon brush, or a sponge. Blend in a circular motion, and finish with downward strokes (to flatten little hairs). Blend at the hairline and jawline. Apply concealer after base – otherwise it can cake or rub off during blending. Dot it on blemishes or dark circles with a small brush, and blend.

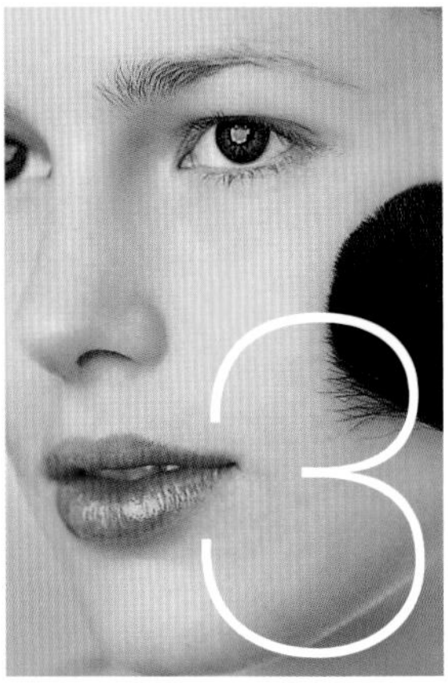

LOCK IT DOWN

Smooth on blush, then powder only oily areas, like the nose and chin. (Women with dry skin can skip this step.) Press a large velvet puff dipped in loose powder gently into the skin, or if you prefer a brush, tap it upright first so the grains settle into the bristles, and sweep over skin in downward strokes.

We've learned how to pick the perfect foundation (even at the drugstore).

Back when we were 11, we made a solemn vow: We would never put that sticky, goopy base stuff on our faces. But just as the males our age have improved considerably since then, so has foundation. New formulas contain silicone powders and light-diffusing pigments to disguise flaws and brighten skin, along with sunscreen and antioxidants to protect it from damage. And since the whole point of base is to even out, not coat, the skin, most are sheer enough to be almost undetectable — except as a smooth, faultless surface.

WHEN CHOOSING A FOUNDATION, first consider your skin's behavior. If you'd like to give your oily face a more matte finish, look for one labeled "oil free," "cream-to-powder," or "mattifying." For combination skin, try a stick foundation, which masks shine in the T-zone. Tinted moisturizer or liquid foundation is perfect for dry skin; if you need more coverage, try a cream or mousse formula (they're usually in small tubs, not bottles).

HERE'S A SIMPLE WAY TO FIGURE OUT YOUR SKIN TONE: If you were out in the sun for an hour without any protection, what would happen? If you would turn bright pink, your skin

probably has a cool tone. (Try ones with "porcelain" or "ivory" in the name.) If it would freckle, tan, or just stay the same (as Asian and African skin often do), then your complexion is warm and needs a yellow-tinged shade ("golden" or "honey" is usually in the name).

SINCE EVEN MAKEUP AT THE DRUGSTORE is often categorized by tone these days, the rest should be a snap. Choose the two or three shades that seem like the best contenders, and draw a stripe of each along your jawline. (If this would involve furtively prying off a tamper-resistant seal, hold the bottle up to your face instead.) Then examine the stripes in natural light, walking straight out of the department store with a hand mirror if necessary; if it's a bottle you're dealing with, head for the nearest window. The right one will seem to disappear into the skin.

IF THE COLOR ISN'T UTTERLY AND EXACTLY PERFECT, you still have options. Several lines offer custom-blended shades, and you can also mix colors together yourself — just be sure to do it on your palm first, not on your face. If you are stuck between two shades, choose the one that's slightly darker. Prepping with moisturizer and adding a dusting of powder can lighten things up.

Trick of the Trade

Applying foundation with a latex sponge makes it easy to see exactly how much you are putting on and aids in blending. Dampen it first, and you end up with slightly more sheer coverage.

Cheater's Guide

Summertime, and the living is . . . greasy. The only thing we hate more than catching sight of our shiny selves in the middle of a hot afternoon is having to wash off all our makeup and start over. Fortunately, there are a few simple steps to minimizing shine all day long.

1 Prep the face with an oil-free moisturizing lotion (for normal or dry skin) or a mattifying lotion (if you tend to get oily).

2 If you can't get away with just concealer, choose a semimatte foundation (look for words like "velvet" or "satin" on the label). Apply base with a damp foam sponge, both to dilute the formula a bit and to avoid depositing extra oil with your fingertips.

3 Set foundation with the least amount of translucent powder possible. Dip a puff in the powder, swirl it on the back of your hand to remove excess, then press onto the nose, chin, and forehead.

4 If powder makes the skin look dry, lightly spritz your face with water or smooth a pea-size dab of highlighting cream over the brow bones and apples of the cheeks to make it more reflective.

5 Perform any touch-ups with a clean puff or blotting papers — not more powder, which will only cake.

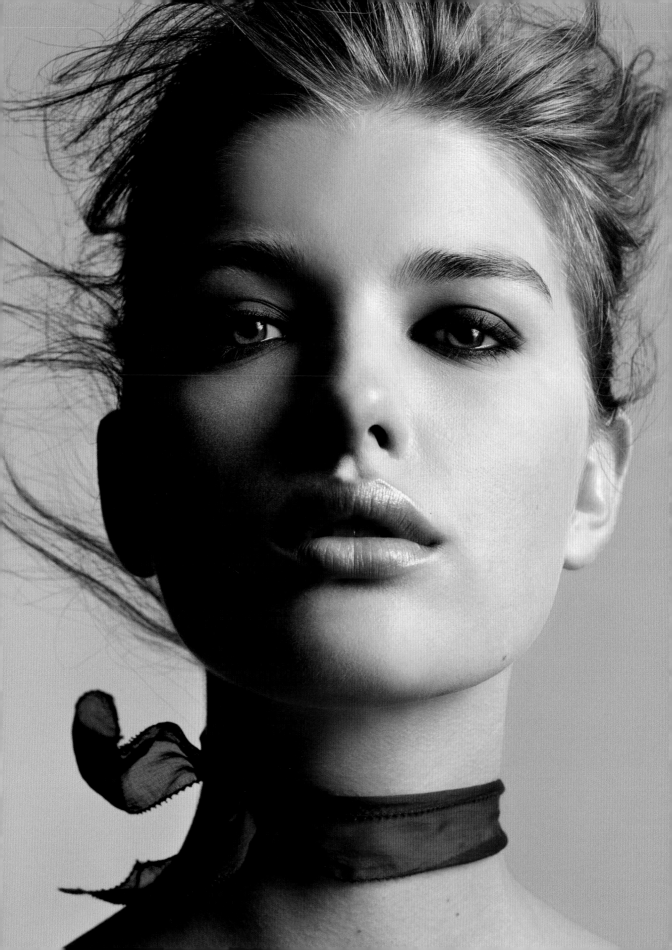

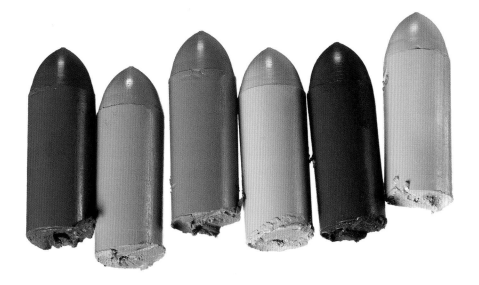

Forget what your narcissistic ex said: Concealer is God's real gift to women.

If we were asked what one makeup product we would choose if stranded on a desert island, concealer just might make the cut (though all that lounging under palm trees would significantly lessen our dark circles).

AS WITH FOUNDATION, you should consider both consistency and color when buying concealer. To see how much coverage it provides, dab some over the blue veins on your wrist. Test the color on the area of your neck just below the ear (since it should be ever so slightly lighter than your foundation).

DON'T GO TOO LIGHT. Concealer that's too pale can turn brown pigment under the eyes a corpselike shade of gray — especially in photographs.

DON'T GO TOO HEAVY, EITHER. If you want concealer to look natural, it's always best to work in thin, sheer layers and build it up gradually. And keep away from the magnifying mirror: Not only do you really not need to see a pimple that close up, but the magnification tends to lead to overapplication.

Trick of the Trade

If you get marooned without your favorite concealer, check the cap of your foundation bottle. The makeup that has collected there is somewhat thicker and perfect for covering up flaws.

Beauty Myth

The Myth: You need a tinted concealer to color-correct certain flaws.

THE TRUTH: We can see why this seemed like a wicked-cool idea back in 1989, since on the color wheel, green does indeed cancel out red. On your face, without expert application, there's a decent chance you'll end up looking like the Incredible Hulk. And experts agree: The color you want in a concealer is the one that most precisely matches your skin.

It took a while, but we've finally conquered our fear of powder.

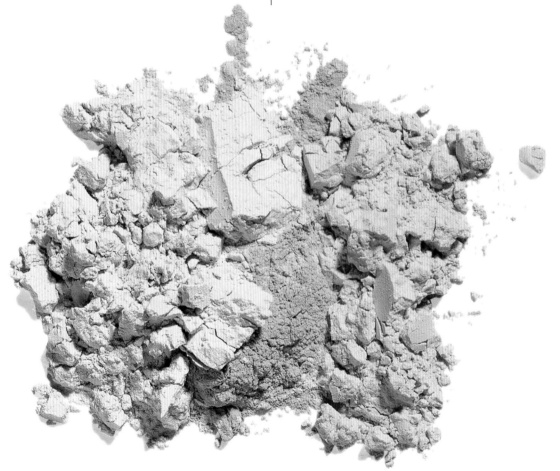

Long after we mastered foundation and concealer, we still resisted the coup de grace: a light dusting of translucent powder that sets the whole look and prevents shine. It sounded simple enough, but the fact remained that it was possible to go from looking elegant to embalmed in one flash of a puff. We now know how to go to the matte.

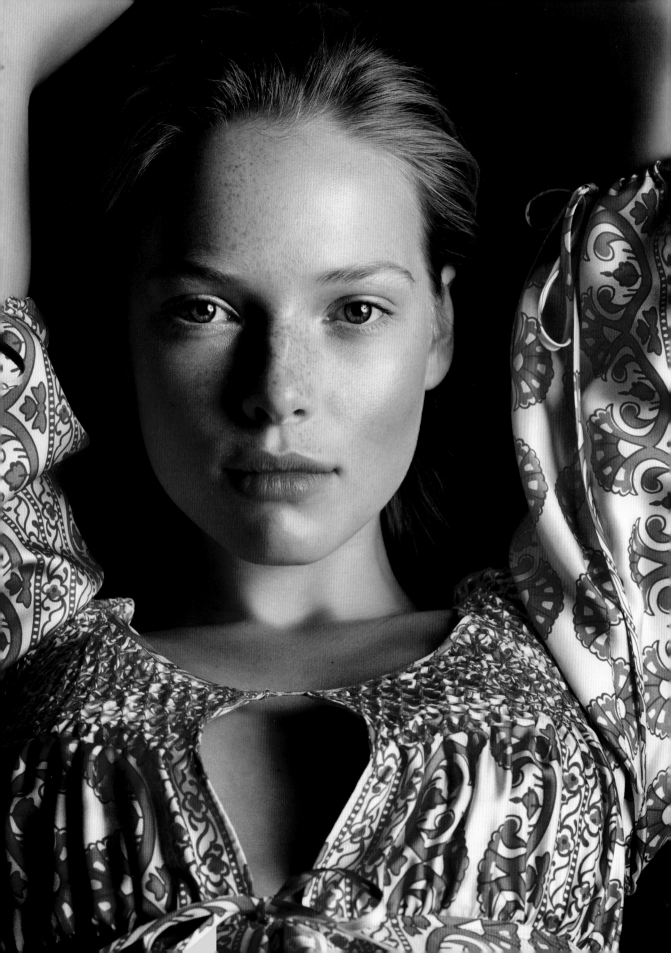

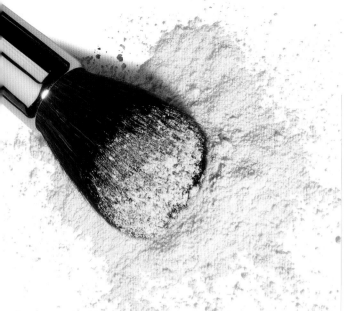

The Art of

The real key to conquering flaws is concealer. A quick overview: "Creamy" means it's typically delivered in a tube, often with a wand or brush attached, and feels (logically enough) like heavy cream. "Cakey" or "thick" concealer is usually dense (the consistency of paste) and sold in a pot, palette, or pan. "Sheer" formulas are liquid; foundation can be used instead in a pinch. Now, on to the battlefield.

Dark circles

Tools: A creamy concealer; a small, flat synthetic brush; sponge; translucent powder

Technique: After dabbing on moisturizer or eye cream and waiting for it to sink in, press concealer into dark areas, using a brush. Start with the inside corners of the eyes and work downward, avoiding the skin right below the bottom lashes (where concealer can make eyes look smaller) and at the outer corners of the eyes (where it accentuates crow's feet). Gently blend the edges with the brush. Set it by patting a few times with a clean, damp sponge, then lightly press a powdered puff over the concealer.

Blemishes

Tools: Q-tip; Visine (or any anti-redness eye drops); cakey concealer; small, flat synthetic brush; translucent loose powder

Technique: Soak a Q-tip in Visine, and place it in the freezer for 30 minutes. Hold it gently on the blemish for a minute to reduce

POWDER IS ABOUT TEXTURE, not color. Rather than choosing a shade that matches or enhances your skin color, it's best to go with a truly translucent formula, which means it has as little pigment as possible.

A LITTLE GOES A LONG WAY. After dipping a large, fluffy brush in powder, give it a vigorous tap against the side of the container, and then apply it just to the T-zone (to control shine). If the resulting look is overly done, experiment — some makeup artists think a big, velvet puff pressed gently into the skin gives the best results.

STAY AWAY FROM THE DANGER ZONES: the inner and outer corners of the eyes and around the mouth. Even a 16-year-old Brazilian model can have powder settle into her smile lines — we've seen it.

THERE ARE TIMES WHEN YOU SHOULDN'T GO ANYWHERE NEAR POWDER. If you have a tan, the odds are that powder will make your skin look gray; consider smoothing a mattifying lotion, which absorbs oil, underneath your makeup, or

Camouflage

redness and swelling, then fan the area dry. Using a brush with a head smaller than the blemish itself, dab a light layer of the pasty concealer on top, then work the brush in a circular pattern to blend slightly around the edges. Let dry, then add one more thin layer. Pat loose powder over the concealer to keep it from budging.

Bruises

Tools: Mauve lipstick; sheer foundation; translucent powder

Technique: Pat just a smidgen of a creamy mauve lipstick over the bruise until it looks pink on the skin. (While we despise those green and lavender concealers, this lipstick trick actually works.) Follow with a layer of foundation over the area, wait a minute, then apply foundation to the entire face. Set with a dusting of translucent powder.

Acne scars

Tools: Cakey concealer; translucent powder

Technique: If the scar is pitted or depressed, choose a concealer that is a shade lighter than your complexion, and use a pointed synthetic brush to fill in the center of the scar without going beyond its edges. If the scar is raised, use your finger to pat on a concealer that matches skin exactly (the warmth of your skin will help it set). Wait a few minutes, then gently press loose powder over the scar a few times with a puff.

Scratches or veins

Tools: Cakey concealer; fine-tipped synthetic brush; translucent powder

Technique: Because scratches are usually both textured and colored, they can be even more difficult to cover than scars. Regular concealer isn't enough; choose an opaque, waterproof formula, then warm a dollop of it by swirling it on the back of your hand. Use the finest makeup brush you have to paint the concealer directly on top of the scratch. The same technique can be used to cover prominent veins, which usually only need one layer; scratches may require two or three. Set by tapping with a finger, then dust lightly with a thin coating of powder.

Trick of the Trade

Many African-American women have skin that is slightly darker on the forehead than on the rest of the face. Don't overcompensate by adding extra layers of makeup elsewhere — use two different shades, and be sure to blend well around the temples and the bridge of the nose.

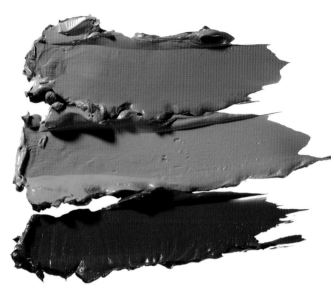

using blotting papers throughout the day instead. On women who have blond facial hair, powder will highlight every last strand; they're better off with a matte-finish foundation. And skip powder altogether on days when you'll be sweating bullets — it is guaranteed to cake on your face. Blotting papers are a better bet.

Never underestimate the power of blush.

According to one recent survey, 59 percent of women wear blush; we'd like to ask the other 41 percent to reconsider. Nothing makes you look healthier than a nice, rosy flush.

GO AHEAD, PINCH YOUR CHEEKS — that's the approximate shade you're looking for. For those with a lower pain tolerance, there are some general guidelines: Light peach or pink looks flattering on fair skin, terra-cotta or apricot warms olive skin, and plum or coral is prettiest on dark tones.

THE VARIOUS FORMULATIONS ALL HAVE THEIR PROS AND CONS. Powder blush can be the most sheer, but also the most difficult to control. Cream formulas blend easily, and many make-up artists say they best mimic the skin's natural flush, but they can aggravate oily or blemished skin. Sheer tints and stains look dewy and soft but are tricky to apply — they dry quickly and require lightning-fast blending (with a sponge, not fingers, to prevent blotchiness).

UNDER NO CIRCUMSTANCE should you be making a fish face when applying blush. Swirl color only on the apples of the cheeks (smile and you'll see them), then blend ever so slightly up and out toward the temples. Think circles, not stripes. And for the most natural look, always start with the tiniest dab of blush, and then build gradually to increase the intensity.

FOR ASIAN WOMEN, an outdoorsy glow depends as much on technique as on color, since the apples of the cheeks are less pronounced.

Beauty 911

The blush that made you look radiant in your dimly lit apartment looks radioactive out on the street.

Don't do the first thing that pops into your panicked head (scrubbing with a tissue will leave a layer of fuzz behind), or the second (makeup remover will only create a streaky mess). Instead, calmly brush a clean cotton ball over your cheeks to remove excess pigment. If that doesn't mute things sufficiently, add a dusting of translucent powder.

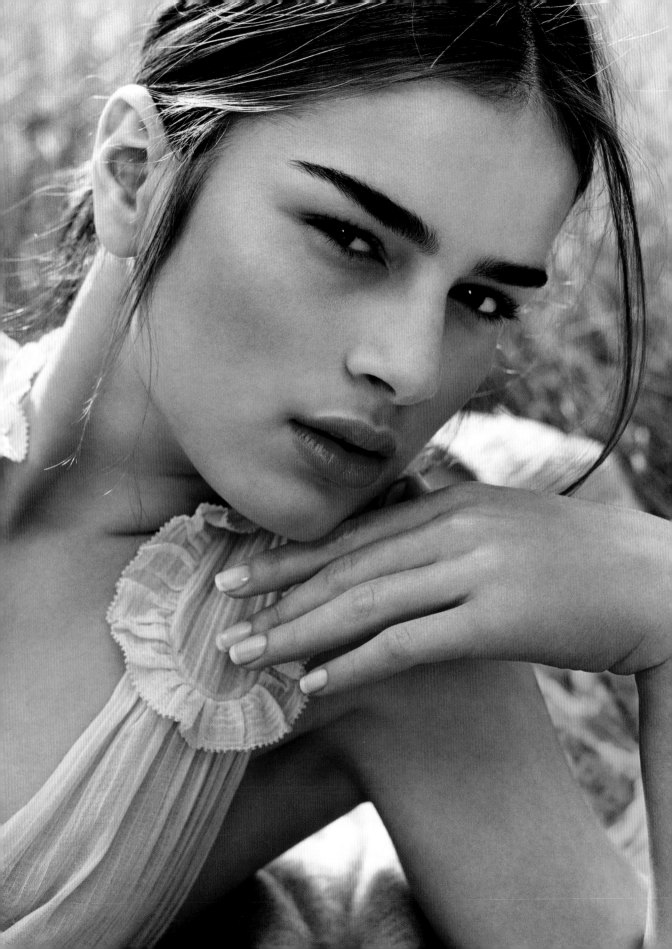

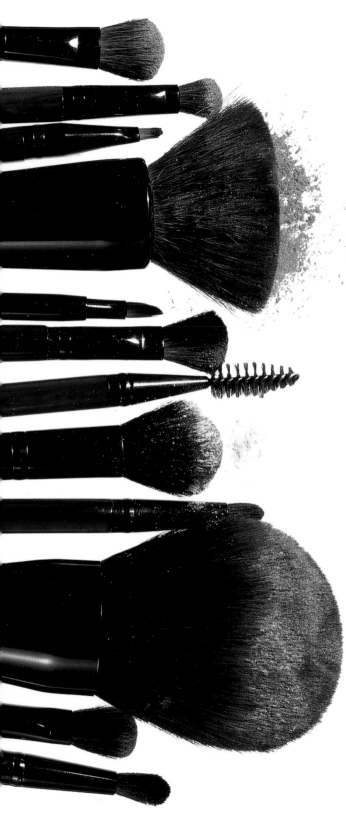

Instead of worrying about them, the pros suggest using just a touch of pastel pink gel or cream blush along and above the cheekbones.

FOR AFRICAN-AMERICAN WOMEN, the idea shouldn't be "blushing" per se, which isn't natural to black skin, but creating a warming effect. Makeup artist Sam Fine suggests starting with a layer of bronzer that's one shade darker than skin, dabbed on with a big brush all over the cheek area, then dusting on a coral or plum powder blush.

We've got our power tools.

Our bathrooms are stocked with a complete set of the most gorgeous sable brushes imaginable, a Christmas gift from a famous makeup artist a few years back. Guests have marveled that the lavish tools look like a work of art, because the majority of them are totally untouched. Here are the trusty old war horses we fall back on.

TWO FLAT, SYNTHETIC BRUSHES FOR CONCEALER. One should be tiny enough that you can dab a thick formula directly onto a blemish without getting the pigment on the surrounding area (as small as one-sixteenth inch); the other, about the size of a pencil eraser and slightly angled, for smoothing on thin layers of creamy undereye concealer. It may sound simpler to use a finger for both, but brushes allow for more precise application and keep you from globbing on too much.

TWO DOME-TIPPED, NATURAL-BRISTLE EYE-SHADOW BRUSHES. According to makeup artist Dick Page, you can pull off just about any look with them. He sold us on the small-headed variety: one a quarter inch wide (for lining the lids and creases), the other a half inch wide (for filling in eyelids or highlighting under the brows).

A 1½-INCH NATURAL-BRISTLE BLUSH BRUSH.
Makeup artist Sue Devitt once declared that this was the ideal size — small enough that you aren't likely to OD on color, big and fluffy enough to blend nicely.

AN OVERSIZE NATURAL-BRISTLE BRUSH FOR LOOSE POWDER. The bigger the better when it comes to whisking excess off the face. Another option — and the one favored by many makeup artists — is using a velvet powder puff.

MAKEUP ARTISTS LOVE NATURAL BRISTLES because they hold an even amount of pigment and distribute it uniformly. (If the prices for sable make you gasp, check out your local art-supply store; they have brushes of comparable quality that are better suited to an MFA's budget.) Just don't use them with anything liquid, which can soak into the bristles and cause them to clog or degrade — that's what those silky white synthetic brushes are for. And as a rule, we try to force ourselves to throw out the skimpy brushes that come in a compact of powder, blush, or eye shadow. They're more likely to have been manufactured to fit the case, not your face.

Guilty as Charged

We rarely wash our makeup brushes.

It would be one thing if we could drop them off at the dry cleaner, but we're more likely to drop them in the garbage (for shame, for shame). It actually takes just a few minutes to wash makeup brushes, and you only need to do it once a month: Grab a bowl, and add one part baby shampoo to four parts water. Swish brushes around, gently separating bristles, and be both gratified and a little horrified by all the pigment that pours out. Rinse thoroughly, and allow brushes to air-dry overnight with the handle resting on a counter and the bristles hanging over the edge. That wasn't so bad, was it?

We love to skip tools entirely and use our fingers.

When we watch makeup artists work backstage at fashion shows, it sometimes looks like finger-painting class at the local preschool (minus the minibottles of Veuve Clicquot, of course). Indeed, there are moments when smearing, smudging, and swiping on your makeup are better than painting it on meticulously with a brush.

HERE'S THE RULE OF THUMB (or forefinger): If the area is larger than your fingertip, go ahead and use it. If it's smaller, pick up a brush.

ANYTHING THAT COMES IN CREAM OR GEL form practically begs to be dabbed on with fingers (which explains why those products never come with an applicator).

BECAUSE OF THE HEAT OF YOUR SKIN, fingers can be the ultimate blending tool, especially for fragile areas like under the eyes. To set concealer over dark circles, lay the pad of your middle or ring finger lightly on top of the skin for 10 or 15 seconds to warm the cover-up and allow it to melt in, then pat around the edges.

We shudder at the mention of the word "contouring."

Back when we were sprawled out on our canopied bed in junior high school, the theory behind contouring made perfect sense: Adding shadows with makeup could change the very look of your bone structure. The reality is that dark streaks on the sides of your nose — or worse, your cheeks — don't make you look chiseled; they make you look dirty. Ironically, the exact opposite approach works wonders: You can use a shimmery highlighting stick, cream, or powder to attract light at points where the sun usually hits the face (rather than shadows where it doesn't). Here's how.

CHOOSE A SHADE: White or silver highlighter is best on fair skin; a slightly bronze one is flattering for dark or olive skin.

PAT OR BRUSH THE HIGHLIGHTER directly on the tops of the cheekbones (over or under blush) and along the brow bones.

IF HIGHLIGHTER SEEMS TOO GLARING ON YOUR SKIN, try this trick we learned from makeup artist Dick Page: Dab a pearlized foundation in a semicircle that starts at the brow bone, goes to the outer corner of the eye, and extends down along the cheekbone. He says it mimics the way light hits the face under the most ideal circumstances (like carefully choreographed photo shoots).

KEEP HIGHLIGHTER FAR AWAY FROM BLEMISHES or anything else you'd prefer not to draw attention to, like fine lines and wrinkles.

There is a dark art to wearing bronzer believably.

Bronzer got a whole lot simpler when we accepted the fact that it isn't supposed to be a portable version of self-tanner. It's actually the summer version of the highlighting techniques outlined above — a way to mimic where the sun falls on the face. A few simple steps can banish any unfortunate associations with pumpkins, alligator handbags, or George Hamilton.

BRONZER SHOULD NEVER BE more than two shades darker than the skin's natural color. Pink- or peach-toned bronzer is best for fair and ruddy skin; copper shades work well with olive skin; and bright, orange copper tones complement dark skin.

TO PREVENT STREAKING, choose cream and gel formulas for dry skin and powders for oily or combination skin. Skip liquid formulas altogether — they can be too drippy and hard to control.

FOR POWDER BRONZER, a blush brush is easier to control than the dinky pad that comes with most compacts. For creams and gels, fingers are best. And regardless of consistency, be sure to blend the bronzer into the skin until there are no discernible lines.

BRONZER IS FOR BONES, not the entire face (unless you are truly pallid, in which case you can dust a very, very thin layer all over). Focus it on the cheekbones, the bones above the temples, the bridge of the nose, and the chin to mimic a natural tan.

FINISH BY SMOOTHING A FAINT LAYER of bronzer down the center of the neck and onto the collarbones to minimize the contrast between your face and everything else.

Shopping for Steals

We've had a perverse fascination with dollar stores ever since we found our favorite discontinued lip liner near the stacks of pork rinds. And every makeup artist we know agrees that if you're going to experiment with teal or tangerine, it's best to start at the 99-cent level. A guide to what to stock up on — and what to avoid at all costs.

POWDERS

Loose powder has the longest shelf life of any makeup, but pressed powder blushes, bronzers, and eye shadow can crumble when broken (hold the package to your ear and shake it before buying). Keep an eye out for department-store "gifts with purchase" — these prizes often show up in dollar stores just a few months after the promotion ends.

LIPSTICK

Made of 95 percent wax, most lipsticks start becoming rancid after three years. Avoid sticks with visible beading, sweating, or a dried-out look — and make sure tubes are stored away from windows or hot lights, which can melt lipstick. Lip gloss is a better bet, as long as the safety seal is intact and the tube is clear (so you can see exactly what shade you are getting).

FOUNDATION

If dermatologists had their way, liquid foundation would be banned from discount-store shelves. Without opening it, there's no way to tell if a bottle has dried out or become rancid. Cream-to-powder formulations are a bit better since they contain less oil, but in time they can shrink from the sides of the pan.

EYE & LIP LINER

Those in plastic tubes often contain silicone, which tends to lose moisture quickly. Wooden pencils are generally fine if they're sealed and the point looks sharp (as further protection, sharpen it before the first use).

TOOLS

Cheap sponges are too porous and tend to suck up makeup, but giant bags of cotton balls and pads are the ultimate bargain — just check the label to make sure they are 100 percent cotton. Makeup artists stay far away from cheap lash curlers (misaligned pads can yank out lashes) and tweezers (which tend not to grab hair well, or tug painfully on skin).

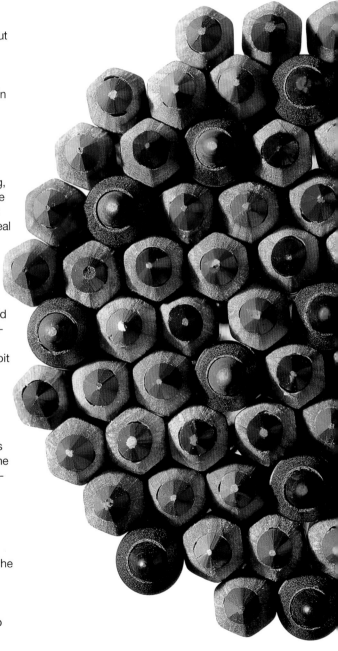

Found in Translation

If we wanted our résumés to be beyond reproach, we'd drop all mention of our farcical college French and replace it with "Fluent in the language of makeup packaging." An abridged dictionary:

"MOISTURIZING," "CREAMY": Will keep dry skin from becoming flaky by the end of the day but make oily complexions look (and feel) even slicker.

"ILLUMINATING," "LINE MINIMIZING," OR "RADIANT": Contains shimmer particles to reflect light from wrinkles. It also, however, will reflect light onto blemishes — skip if your skin isn't clear.

"CREAM-TO-POWDER," "MATTIFYING": Dries to a powdery finish that's ideal for very oily skin; far too *What Ever Happened to Baby Jane?* for dry skin.

"TINT" OR "GEL": The color is definitely sheer — and it will probably fade fast.

"STAIN": Light, sheer, and not the least bit shiny. Also known for drying fast and fading slowly.

"LONG WEARING," "ENDURING," OR "LASTING": Intensely pigmented formulas designed to cling to the skin. (Antonym: "sheer.")

Trick of the Trade

Be wary of foundations that look pink in the bottle — they make skin disturbingly rosy (think Miss Piggy). The slightest tint of yellow, while not as appealing in the bottle, is actually more universally flattering and helps neutralize any redness in your face.

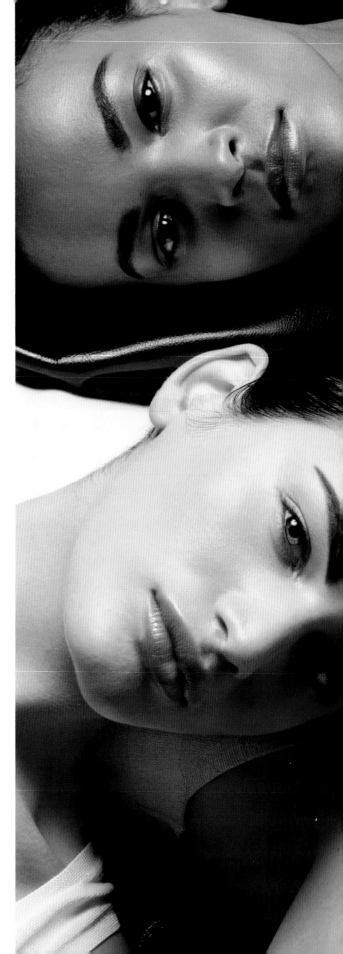

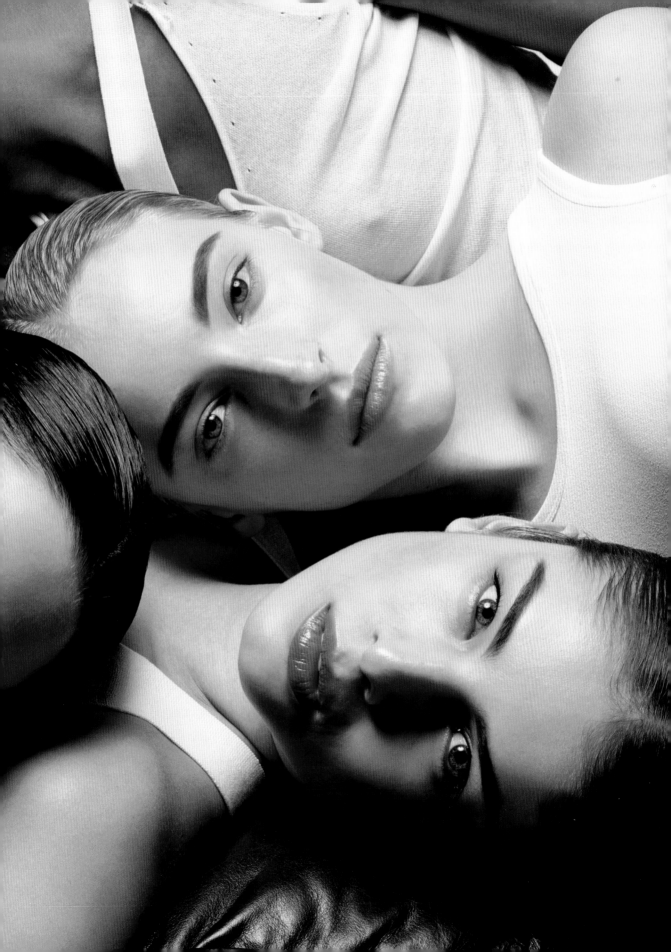

The 10 Commandments

1
Always dab on moisturizer or primer before foundation.

2
Test foundation on your jawline — not your hand — to find the perfect match.

3
Choose a thin concealer for undereye circles and a pasty one to cover zits.

4
Except for cover-up, makeup should be as sheer as possible.

5
Invest in good-quality brushes (you only need a few).

6
Don't be afraid to apply color with your fingers.

7
Blush should go on the apples of the cheeks, not in the hollows.

8
Highlighter can accentuate your bone structure, but use it sparingly.

9
A little translucent loose powder goes a long way.

10
For a truly natural look, blend, blend, blend.

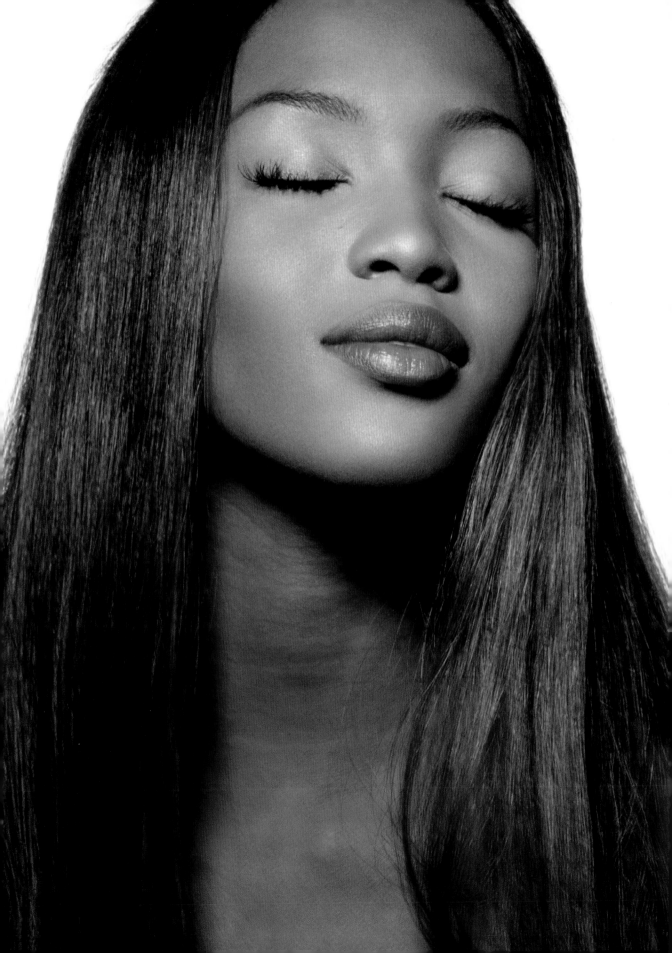

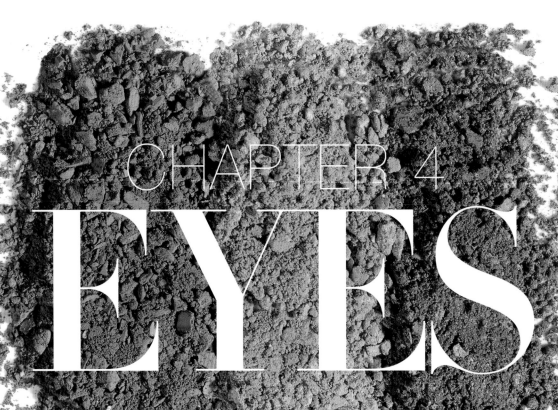

CHAPTER 4

EYES

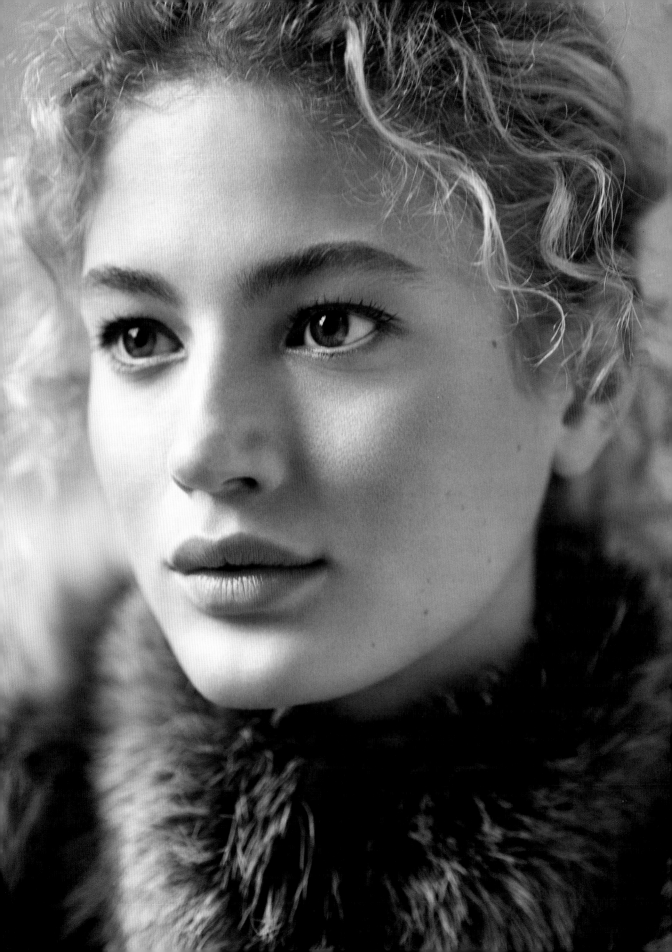

Despite all I've learned about makeup, I've rarely changed my own basic look from season to season, or even year to year. This bewilders colleagues, who have been known to whisper, "You realize, Linda doesn't wear makeup."

Of course, I do wear makeup. I also visit a manicurist, a dermatologist, a star hairstylist, even a brow groomer every few weeks. But you'd hardly know it, or at least that's the goal. While I slather on gallons of products, my aim is to look as if I've exerted no effort, as if I were the rarest of creatures: a natural beauty.

Since I harbor no illusions of being a beauty queen, I decided, for a few weeks one spring, to give up the pretense of naturalness, too. My accomplice was an Italian hair and makeup artist, Letizia Maestri, who came to my hotel every morning before the fashion shows, first in Milan and then in Paris. Letizia's visits were intended to get me camera-ready for TV interviews. But I had a hidden agenda.

Letizia doesn't speak much English; I don't speak Italian, and this became key to our experiment. At my first meeting with most makeup artists, I launch into a list of prohibitions: no pencils, no strong colors, no red lips, no sparkle. Sorry. When Letizia arrived at my room every morning, I offered her a cup of cappuccino and my freshly washed face. When she snapped open her eye-shadow palette and started humming, I did my best to seem nonchalant. She stuck a black pencil smack into my eye and skimmed it along the inner lids while I blinked uncontrollably, something I'd warned readers against for years. She dipped her brush first in a color that resembled the dust on a chocolate truffle, and then in gold and peach powder. Letizia offered commentary, unintelligible to me. "*Che carina,*" she said, stepping back to admire her work. When she handed me a mirror, I tried not to gasp.

I felt absurd and conspicuous, like some mad diva, as I took my seat at the shows. Among the fashion crowd, the only thing worse than neglect is obvious, diligent enterprise. With my shadowed, smoked, lined, and highlighted eyes, there was no question that I'd tried hard to look good, or to look like someone else — Maria Callas? Mariah Carey? I wasn't sure.

"Today, we make you a French lady," Letizia announced when we moved the operation to Paris. "A French lady" apparently wears gray and black eye shadows and a potent chestnut lipstick. It sounds awful, and it may have been, but I'd lost all perspective. Before I left the hotel room one day, Letizia looked me over and frowned theatrically. "You are like the man," she said, and ordered me into the bathroom to put on fragrance. Then she hauled out a can of body-makeup mousse and squirted it on my legs. All day, I felt unspeakably glamorous. People stopped me to compliment my extraordinary eye makeup. They may have been mocking me, but I thanked them just the same.

When my stint with Letizia ended, I returned to doing my own eyelash curling and lip glossing. Perhaps I won't miss the gold powder, but that brief dose of glamour has left me questioning my insistence on a natural, effortless look that is neither of the two. Sometimes there's less vanity, and more honesty, in showing a little effort.

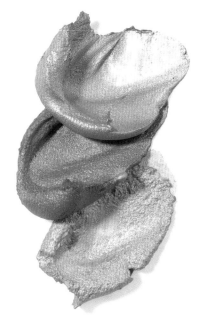

We've finally figured out where all those shadow colors are supposed to go.

Like ocean waves and blind mice, eye shadows always seem to come in threes. We have no explanation for the rodent thing, but beauty companies package colors (like bone, taupe, and brown) together to take the guesswork out of eye makeup for you. Here's how to use them.

THE MINIMUM: Before we get to the colors, don't forget to prime your lids with a dab of foundation or loose translucent powder. Then dust the lightest shadow shade over the entire lid, from the lash line to the brow, to brighten the eyes. This could be all the eye shadow you need.

THE MIDDLE GROUND: Choose a shadow with a touch of the color that complements your eyes, like chestnut or mahogany for green eyes, gray or lavender for blue eyes, and any color for brown eyes, as long as the shadow is darker or paler than the iris itself. Apply this second shade from the lashes to a point just past the crease, and blend lightly.

THE MAXIMUM: The darkest shade lines the lashes (either alone, or on top of pencil). Dampen a small, angled brush with hard bristles, and dunk it into a little powder. Get the brush as close to the lash line as possible. When you're finished, sweep away any stray shadow that has fallen onto the cheeks.

Trick of the Trade

Always apply liner before mascara. The pressure of your hand (especially while you're concentrating so hard on drawing that perfect line) can cause the lashes to stick together or the mascara to smear.

Beauty Myth

The Myth: Your eye shadow should match your eye color.

THE TRUTH: What a dreary thought — only being able to wear one color of shadow for life. Besides being monotonous, matching your makeup to your eye color can look tacky (blue eyes + blue shadow = Smurfette). Instead, choose a shade that creates contrast: for example, mahogany for green eyes, violet for blue eyes, and gold for brown eyes. With a little experimentation, you'll figure out what looks most striking on you.

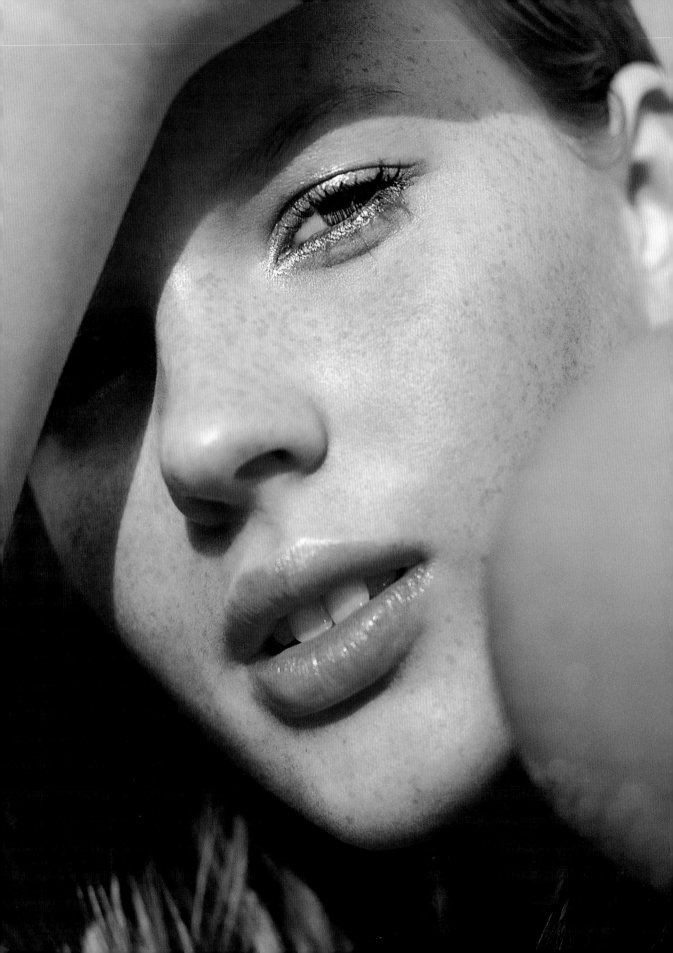

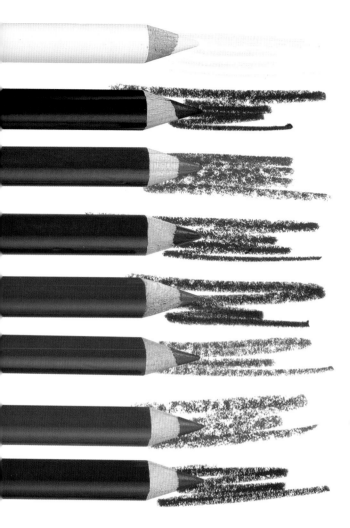

khaki) will highlight green eyes; lighter browns with a slight golden or gray tinge (sand or taupe) flatter blue eyes; and those with brown peepers should look for a dark, almost charcoal brown to avoid matching their eye color exactly.

ANOTHER ADVANTAGE TO BROWN: It can create a smoky look without seeming garish or Goth. Take a medium brown shade and sweep it all over the lids (to just above the crease). Then fan the color outward ever so slightly toward the temples. Those who are daunted by eyeliner can tap the very tip of a stiff, flat brush into a darker shade, then stipple it right up against the lash line.

And we've mastered eyeliner. Next up, quantum physics . . .

Just as the Wonderbra enhances the bustline, eyeliner can make even the smallest eyes look bigger. And just like choosing between nude Lycra and black lace, you've got several options.

WE GENERALLY STICK TO PENCIL, considering that even many professional makeup artists are afraid of liquid liner. Thin and precise works for day (when we want the effect to be subtle); chubby and smudged, at night. Basic black or brown is always a safe bet, but don't be afraid to experiment with muted colors. Navy or slate gray is amazing on blue eyes; rich hunter green and deep purple enhance brown eyes; and chocolate liner makes green eyes look even brighter.

APPLY LINER ACCORDING TO your eye shape. If you have close-set eyes, draw it only at the outer corners. Otherwise, line the entire upper lid. With one hand, lift the eyelid by pushing up on the brow bone, and with the other, draw small dashes along your top

When in doubt, we choose brown.

The answer to that question squawking out of the TV — "What can brown do for you?" — seems perfectly clear to us. Because even the fairest skin has some amount of brown in it, it's almost impossible for cocoa eye shadow to look unnatural in the way that, say, just about any blue can.

OF COURSE, heading to the cosmetics department and asking for brown shadow will yield as many hues as browsing for white paint at the Home Depot. If you need a little direction, consider that shades with yellow undertones (like

lashes from the inner corner outward. (If you want to make eyes look wider, extend the liner a millimeter or two beyond the corner.)

MAKE SURE NO SKIN SHOWS between the line and the lash roots. If this escapes you, forget about drawing a line, and instead wedge the point of the pencil right at the roots of the lashes, making tiny dots every few hairs. (This is a trick we learned from Laura Mercier, and it's a good one for the liner-phobic.)

IF YOU WANT TO BRAVE LIQUID LINER, don't bother painting on one continuous line. Dab on equally spaced dots starting at the inner corner — a total of four or five in all — then go back and connect them. Blend quickly with a Q-tip to blur the borders, or brush over the liquid liner with matching powder shadow, a trick that also makes the line look less severe.

Guilty as Charged

We line the inner rims of our eyes.

We've been lectured against it by some of the top ophthalmologists in the world. But we can't help it: We love the way eyeliner looks on the inner rims. The practice, while not exactly dire, raises the risk of infection and other unpleasantness. Doctors suggest minimizing the risk by sharpening your eye pencil before every use (and cleaning the sharpener itself with alcohol every week or so).

Smoky Eyes 101

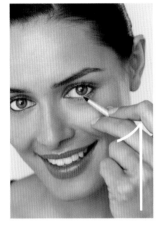

LINE LIDS

With a sharpened, soft black pencil, start at the inner corners of the upper lashes, and draw small, diagonal downward strokes. Rub a clean Q-tip or sponge-tip applicator over the liner, smudging it halfway up the lids. Then, with short strokes, draw liner just at the outer edges of the lower lashes, and smudge slightly.

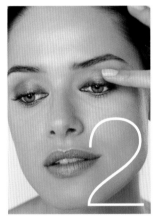

ADD SHADOW

With your ring finger, apply a cream shadow in a pale silver or metallic gray over the lids and up to the brow bone. Smudge it about an eighth inch toward the temples. Brush a slightly darker gray or silver powder shadow over that, blending so it fades right above the crease.

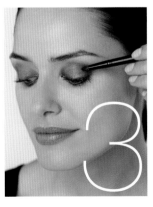

DEFINE EYES

Curl the top lashes, and coat them with a few layers of black mascara. Keep the rest of your makeup light, but not ghostly, by smoothing on a berry or nude lipstick and a faint pink or rose blush.

We're pros at picking the right mascara — without even opening up the tube.

You know how you aren't supposed to judge a book by its cover? Feel free to go ahead and judge mascara by its label: Cosmetics companies have code words that convey the overriding goal of each formula.

"EXTEND," "LENGTHENING," AND "FIBERS" all mean the mascara will make your lashes look longer. (One warning: Fibers can fall into the eyes during the day and get stuck under contact lenses.) The brush inside is usually conical or cylindrical, with tight bristles.

"MAXIMUM," "VOLUMIZING," "BUILDING," and "thickening" mean your lashes will look fatter. The brush here is slightly rigid, with well-spaced bristles that will deposit the most pigment.

WHEN YOU WANT IT ALL — long, thick lashes that almost look fake — pick a mascara with some variation of the word "fake" in the name ("false," "fantasy," "faux") and a large, full brush that's dense in the middle and has a tapered tip.

FOR A NATURAL LOOK, avoid volumizers, thickeners, and fibers, and search for words like "basic" or "tint." The brush isn't as important in this case — just be sure to clean it often to prevent clumps.

Applying mascara is not as simple as you'd think.

Swipe, swipe, done — right? Wrong. In the immortal words of rappers 2 in a Room, "wiggle it just a little bit."

IF YOU WANT THICK LASHES without clumps, start with a white or translucent primer (sometimes packaged at the other end of a mascara tube). One coat helps mascara go on smoothly.

YOU KNOW THAT GUNK THAT COLLECTS at the tip of the mascara wand? It's as messy as bubblegum. Never scrape it against the mouth of the tube, which only causes large, dry clumps to form. Squeeze the wand in a paper towel instead.

WEDGE THE BRUSH RIGHT NEAR the roots of the lashes, and wiggle it back and forth. Not only will this make the lashes look fuller, but it also functions as eyeliner.

CONSIDER DOUBLING UP. Lots of makeup artists work with more than one formula at a time, starting with a mascara that has a fat brush,

Beauty Myth

The Myth: Pumping your mascara wand will rid it of clumps.

THE TRUTH: All that pumping the wand does is fill the tube with air — making the formula dry out faster and clump more. After those first few silky swipes, it's inevitable that pigment will start to cling to the brush. The only foolproof solution is to wipe down the wand with a paper towel (which leaves less lint than tissue) before each application.

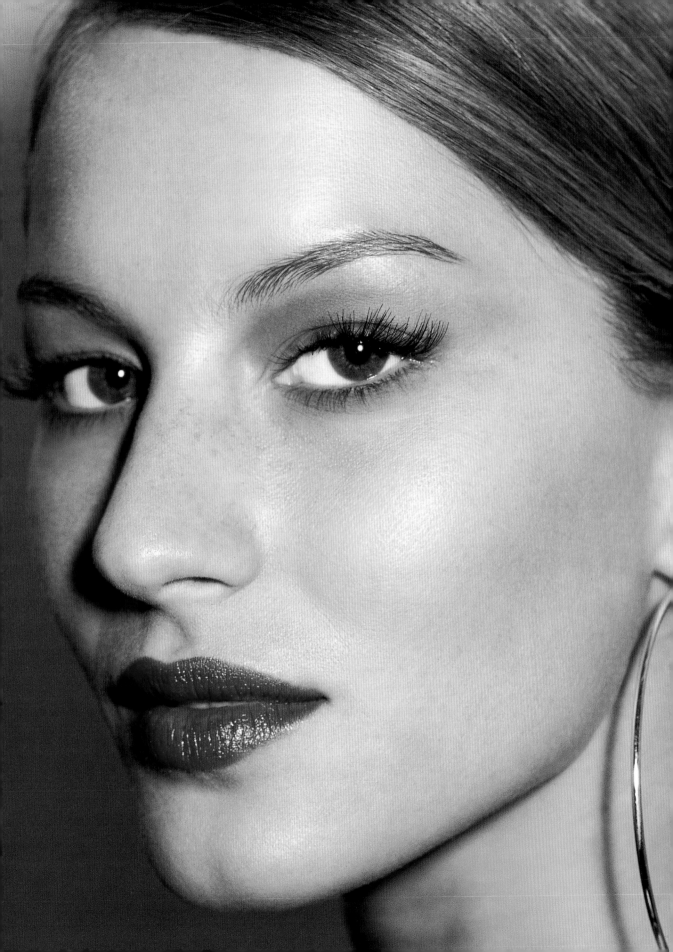

sweeping all the way to the tips, then following with a skinny-brushed mascara, holding it vertically (like a windshield wiper) and sweeping it back and forth through lashes to catch every last hair — especially at the corners.

ON LOWER LASHES, keep mascara to a minimum. It veers too easily into spider-leg territory and casts a dark shadow under your eyes (and who needs that?).

If they banned eyelash curlers from commercial flights, we'd consider taking the train.

It's an initiation ritual for beauty editors: Those who saw *A Clockwork Orange* have become desensitized to clamping metal near their eyes. It's worth it: With just a few squeezes, a curler makes lashes look longer and eyes appear wider.

BUY A HIGH-QUALITY CURLER, and you'll have it for ages. The trick is to find one that matches the curve of your eyes: The more deep-set they are, the rounder the curler should be. And if you have trouble reaching the inner or outer corners, consider an individual-lash curler (it's a quarter the size of a regular model).

FOR A NATURAL CURL, gently squeeze for ten seconds: first near the roots, then in the middle of

the lashes, and finally right near the tips. There's no need to pinch the curler over and over; lashes are fragile and don't appreciate the agitation.

IF YOUR LASHES LOSE THEIR CURL as the day progresses, consider adding heat to the mix. Run a metal curler under hot water for 30 seconds, dry it off, and test it against your forearm to make sure it isn't too hot. Tempting as it may be, heating things up with a blow-dryer can easily lead to burns.

BE SURE TO MAINTAIN YOUR TOOL: Replace the rubber tip of the curler every six months, or whenever it seems to stop curling effectively.

We've learned how to keep our eye makeup from going AWOL.

A few steps can prevent shadow, liner, and mascara from disappearing into thin air.

EYE SHADOW CREASES when the natural oils in the skin mix with pigments and collect in the folds of the upper lids. Prime skin with a dab of concealer or foundation first, and follow with a dusting of translucent powder before applying powder shadow. Keep in mind that strong shades and cream formulas crease more noticeably than neutral powder ones.

Beauty Myth

The Myth: You have to curl lashes before you apply mascara.

THE TRUTH: We once solicited readers for their favorite beauty tricks, and one told us she always curled her lashes after applying mascara because it helped the bend last all day. We followed her advice and got hooked. The trick is to wait at least five minutes for the mascara to dry so that lashes don't end up sticking to the curler and getting yanked out.

Optical Illusions

Not everyone was born with huge, perfectly shaped eyes. That doesn't mean you can't look as if you were.

TO MAKE EYES APPEAR LARGER, add a soft wash of color to the lids all the way up to the brow bones — a very pale pink on pale skin, beige on medium skin, and taupe for dark skin. Then, rather than lining the entire eye with a dark pencil, which can make eyes look smaller, dot white or beige liner between the bottom lashes, and use a skinny brush to smudge gray or brown shadow along the upper lash line only.

TO MAKE CLOSE-SET EYES APPEAR WIDER, lighten the area nearest the nose. With a tiny brush, dab a bit of white, slightly shimmery cream in the area between the inner corners and the nose, then blend.

TO BRING WIDE-SET EYES CLOSER TOGETHER, apply the deepest colors — both shadow and liner — to the half of the eye near the nose, then blend toward the outer corners until the color fades away to nothing.

TO GIVE EYES MORE DEPTH, sweep the lids with a pale taupe or beige shadow, then tuck a light brown or gray into the crease with an angled brush. Blend the two shades well with a soft brush, then smudge just a bit of highlighting cream onto the brow bones for contrast.

Trick of the Trade

If lashes become clumped with mascara, go over them with a clean spooley brush — makeup artists say it's more effective at separating than those little metal combs. In a pinch, the corner of a matchbook works, too.

CRASH COURSE

Fake Lashes

Back in college, we swore to our friends that we'd never fake it. Now that we've been around the block a few times, we realize that we're willing to make an exception to this rule — if just for one night. Here's how to make fakes look as natural as possible.

1 Choose clusters of individual lashes, not a full band. Find ones that are the same length as your natural lashes, or trim them with eyebrow scissors, snipping a tiny bit off each lash (at an angle) so they're slightly different lengths. Reserve the longest clusters for the outer corners of the eyes.

2 Before attaching the fakes, curl your own lashes, and line your eyes with a dark brown or black pencil. This will help conceal the lash roots.

3 Put a drop of lash glue on a hard surface, like the outside of the case the lashes came in, and let it dry for a minute, until it's tacky. Hold the lash tip with tweezers, and dip the root in the glue.

4 Starting at the outer corners, wedge the glued end between your natural lashes, and hold it in place for a few seconds. A couple of clusters at the outer corners of the upper lashes are usually enough, but you can also use them to fill in sparse areas. For the most natural effect, don't glue on more than five clusters to each eye, and steer clear of the inner corners.

5 Once lashes are set, apply shadow and a few coats of mascara to blend the fakes with your natural ones. To remove, wet lashes with water or an oil-based makeup remover — that should be enough to soften the glue.

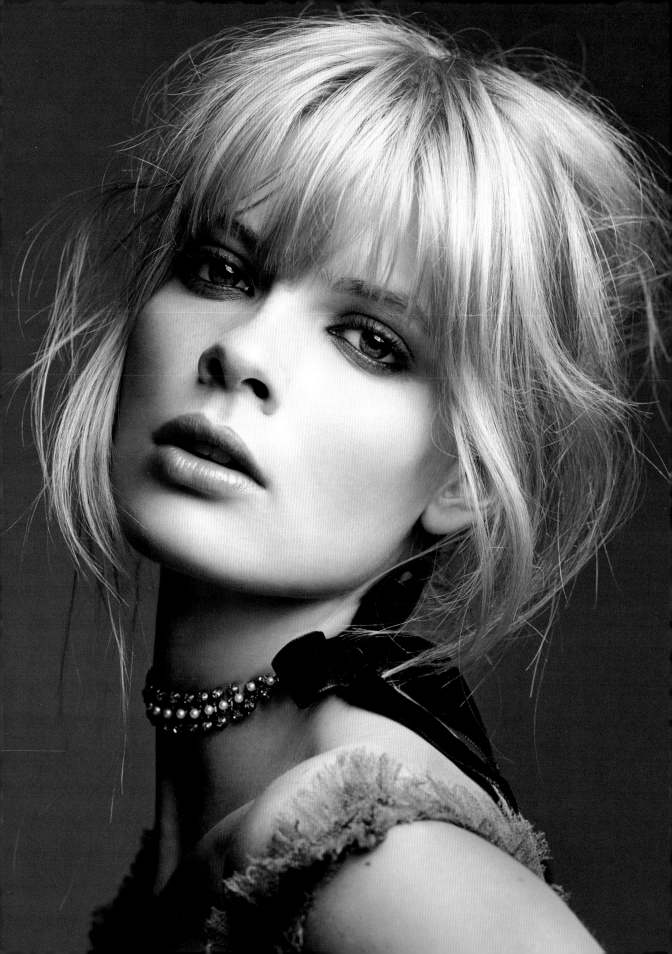

LIQUID LINER USUALLY STAYS IN PLACE all day, but it's also a real challenge to apply. Instead, choose a waterproof pencil or one that contains an ingredient called nylon-12, which won't smudge or fade away. Then set the pencil with a matching powder shadow, pressing it into the liner with a stiff, angled brush.

WATERPROOF MASCARA stands up to an emotional day or a humid night, but it can also flake easily and irritate contact lenses. Makeup artists recommend choosing formulas that contain beeswax, because they tend to be more malleable. Or look for a tube labeled "water resistant" — you can't wear it in the ocean and expect miracles, but it'll be easier to get off and won't run unless you rub it.

We may be exhausted, but at least we don't look it.

There's nothing quite as infuriating as a smirking co-worker asking, "Heyyyyy, rough night?" We've learned to at least *look* as if we got a full eight hours of beauty sleep.

NOTHING SAYS, "Why, yes, I was there at last call," like bloodshot eyes, which are usually caused by dehydration (the source of most hangover misery). A few moisturizing eye drops when you wake up and around lunchtime should help. Experts warn against whitening drops, because they can create rebound redness once you stop using them. But if you look like the crazed villain from a comic book, it won't hurt to try them for a day.

AFTER APPLYING CONCEALER to the all-but-inevitable dark circles, check to see if you need to pat some on your upper lids as well — blood vessels may be visible through the delicate skin. Ditto with the hollow between the bridge of the nose and the inner corner of the eye; turn your face 45 degrees from the mirror, and check for shadows.

A LITTLE SHIMMER CAN CREATE a trompe l'oeil effect. Take a white or beige eye pencil, and draw it along the inner rims of the lower lids (which tend to look red when you're tired). Then sweep a little highlighting cream or powder on the brow bones and in those hollows next to the nose to brighten the whole eye area. The rest of your eye makeup should be minimal — a neutral shadow on the lids and curled mascara.

Cheater's Guide

When we don't have the time or inclination to do full-on eye makeup before going out at night, we use a trick we learned from makeup artist Gucci Westman. Dip your finger in a pot of waxy lip balm, then scribble a little dark brown or black eyeliner on top of the balm. Gently rub the finger into the roots of the top lashes, and finish with several thick coats of mascara. The result is very rock star, and the more it smears the better it looks — no touch-ups necessary.

Trick of the Trade

To keep an eye-shadow application from devolving into a mess, fold a tissue into quarters, and wedge it under your lower lashes while dusting on color. Any errant wisps of pigment will fall onto the paper instead of your skin.

We exercise restraint in the presence of tweezers.

Eyebrows can make or break a face — and don't come off with soap and water.

CONSIDER HAVING YOUR BROWS PLUCKED or waxed by a pro at least once; you can then follow that shape when performing home maintenance.

IF YOU WANT TO SHAPE YOUR OWN BROWS, the general guidelines are as follows: Place a pencil vertically against one nostril — the spot where the pencil meets the forehead is where the brow should begin. Then angle the pencil so it crosses from the center of the bottom lip to the iris — that should be the upper point of the arch. For the brow's end, angle the pencil from the center of the lower lip to the outer corner of the eye. Mark these points with an eye pencil.

WITH A SLANT-HEAD TWEEZER, yank out any strays below the brow line, hair by hair (tweezing clusters can create bald spots). To keep the arches symmetrical, switch from one brow to the other after every three or four hairs, and step back from the mirror to check your progress. Standing too close — or worse, using a magnifying mirror — will lead to trouble. Stop before you've gone too far; it's better to pluck too little than too much.

THE FINAL STEP in getting that perfect curve is the scariest: trimming. Brush each brow straight up with a spooley brush (a spiral-bristled brush that looks like a mascara wand), then press the brush against the brow. Trim any hairs that stick up past the brush with straight (not curved) nail scissors. Repeat on the other brow. If this makes you nervous, just skip it.

There's the Joan Crawford way to fill brows, and then there's our way.

Ever since makeup artist Dick Page told us that he'd never worked on a model who didn't need to have her eyebrows filled in, we've paid more attention to that makeup step.

PENCILS ARE EASY TO USE, portable, and available in every color you might possibly need (for dark brows, a shade lighter than your own brow color will blend in best; for pale brows, go a shade darker). You want to draw on tiny, individual hairs, not a continuous line, and that requires a sharp pencil.

MANY MAKEUP PROS FAVOR brow powder because it looks most natural, especially on fair hair. And brow creams look nice because they are as shiny as the little hairs themselves. Dab either with a small, angled brush in short strokes.

Beauty 911

Your brows have giant divots where you overplucked.

Put down your tweezers, and vow not to pick them up until the hair has grown back. In the meantime, use a thin, flat-edged brush to dab brow powder that's a shade lighter (or darker, if brows are pale) than yours exactly into the holes, starting at the bottom edge and working your way up. To help brows grow back, dab men's extra-strength Rogaine on the area with a Q-tip twice a day for up to four months. Just be careful not to let it drip anywhere near your eyes.

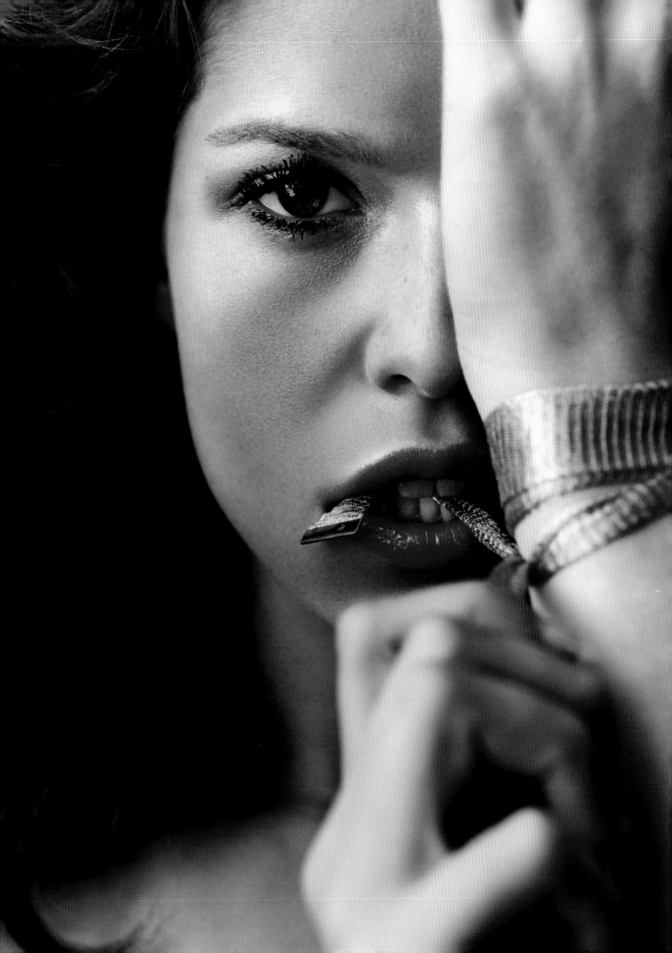

The 10 Commandments

1
To keep eye makeup from disappearing, prime the lids with a little foundation or translucent powder.

2
There is a shade of brown eye shadow that works on everyone.

3
To brighten eyes, apply a pale neutral shadow with a bit of shimmer.

4
Eyeliner and shadow should go on before mascara.

5
Line eyes with pencil, not liquid, in small strokes to keep from making a mess.

6
Don't let any skin show between your lashes and your liner. Use a Q-tip to smudge the line.

7
Curling the eyelashes makes eyes look bigger and lashes look longer.

8
Don't merely comb: Wiggle the mascara brush right at the base of the lashes.

9
Get a professional to groom your brows at least once to determine their best shape.

10
All brows need to be filled in with a little pencil or powder — just don't overdo it.

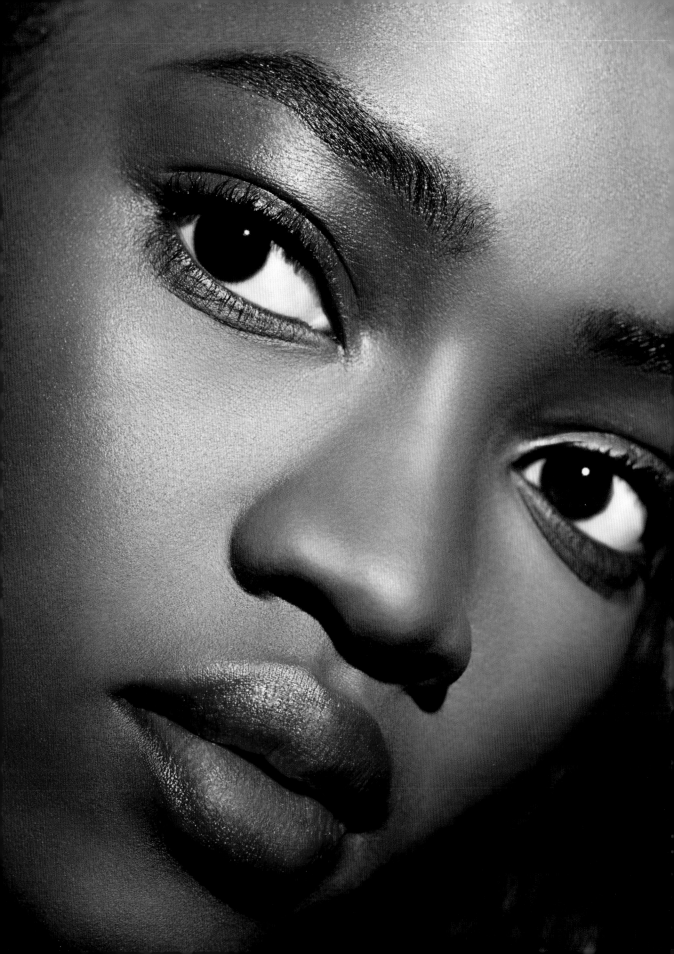

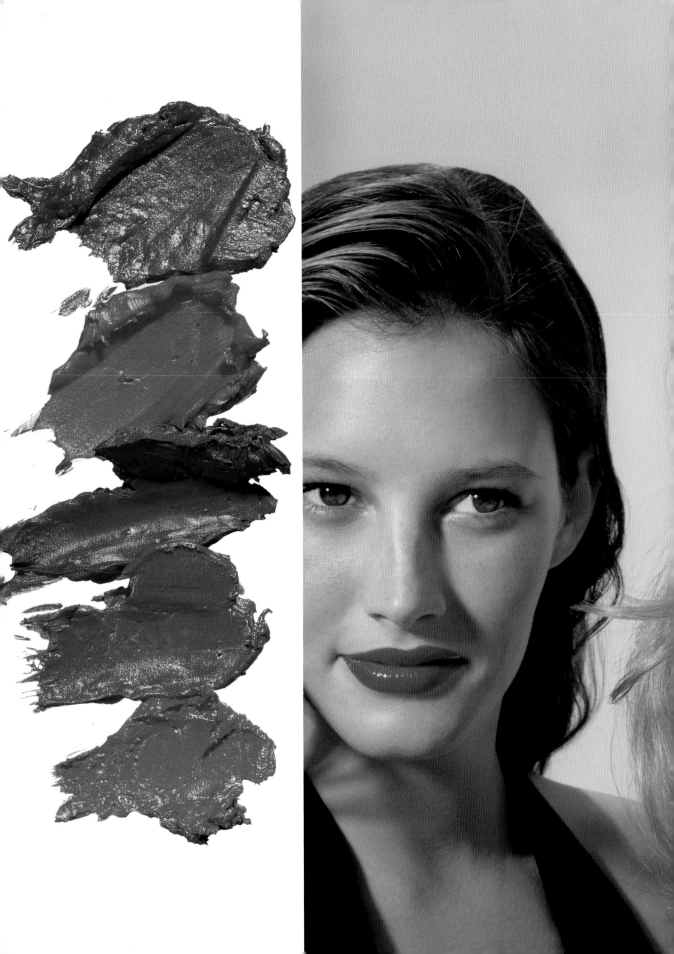

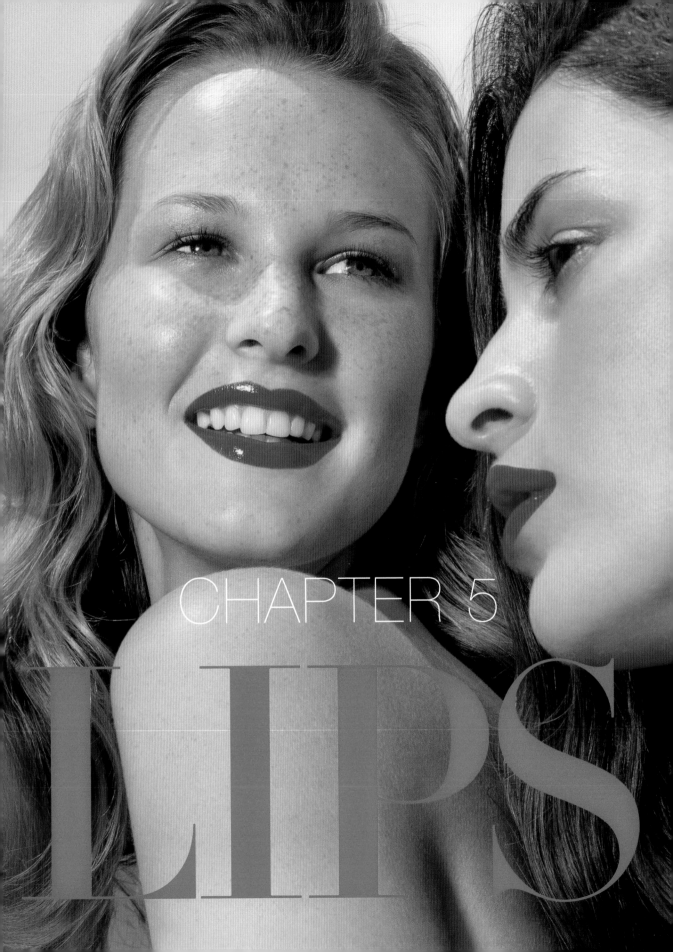

CHAPTER 5

LIPS

I got my first makeup lesson back in the late 1980s from Bobbi Brown. This was before she was rich and famous, before she had her own line of products, back when people still confused her with the guy who sang "My Prerogative." We sat at a table in her boyfriend's apartment, where she showed me how to blow on an eye-shadow brush before skimming it over my lids and to swirl blush on the apples of my cheeks. I still use those tricks.

Before I left, she pressed a tube of lipstick into my hand as if she were giving me an ancient talisman. The plastic case was cracked, the bullet was worn down to a nub, but the fleshy pink shade was as close to perfect as anything I'd ever seen.

I was careful to dip into the lipstick only on special occasions and apply it parsimoniously with a tiny brush. I gave a precious chunk of it to a man who boasted that his company could copy any color in creation. Months later, a box holding three new lipsticks arrived at my office. What a disappointment. The laboratory had added a large dose of frost that gave my beloved color a strange ashen cast.

I've been searching fairly regularly for a replacement ever since I scraped the last bit from that old tube. Every day I carry with me eight lip glosses that rattle around in the bottom of my bag. All have their merits and appeal, but one is too pink, another is too taupe, and a third veers dangerously close to terra-cotta. None is the one.

I've tried to move on. I switched to a slash of bright crimson, which I wore with a Valentino gown to a benefit in Los Angeles one evening. Celebrities stood onstage and told moving tales of hardship, Willie Nelson sang about all the girls he'd loved before, but all I could think about was rubbing that red pigment off my lips. I was sure it had seeped onto my teeth and beyond the corners of my mouth, and that the paparazzi would mistake me for Courtney Love on a bender.

I know the ideal shade is out there; all I have to do is find it. Every time I walk into Saks or Sephora, I feel a flutter of hope, which may be why I keep looking. The search for perfection — elusive, tantalizing — is almost as gratifying as the achievement.

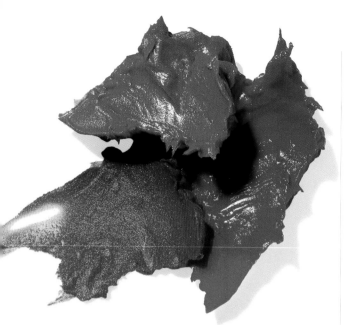

Cheater's Guide

Seventy-nine percent of women wear lip color, according to one recent study. We suspect that at any given time, half of them are probably in front of the mirror making touch-ups. Here's how to slap on a little color without much thought — or time.

1 If eating is on the agenda, consider saturating lips with a liquid stain or long-wearing lipstick, allowing it to dry for a minute, then finishing with a sheer gloss in the same shade. Gloss is less annoying to reapply surreptitiously, and your base color won't desert you by dessert.

2 Ever wonder what those extra-skinny lipsticks are for? Finishing touches in the back of a cab — no mirror required.

3 If touch-ups are truly out of the question, consider just patting on some lip balm and amping up the eyes instead. It looks just as polished — and smoky eye makeup doesn't wear off as quickly.

Eureka, we have found it (the perfect lip color, that is).

The "I'm not wearing any makeup" makeup look we usually favor requires the subtlest of lip color. We like the way makeup artist Dick Page explains the perfect shade (in that cute English accent of his): "Think of your mouth color after a good snog — it's usually a rosy shade that's not too brown." To find it, test shades by covering half your mouth with lipstick and leaving the other half bare. If the lipstick side is the same tone as the naked side but slightly deeper and glossier, then you've nailed it.

Beauty 911
Your lipstick isn't just bleeding; it's hemorrhaging.

Wipe off your entire mouth with a damp tissue or paper towel (if it's an extremely dark or matte shade, a nonoily makeup remover will work better). Then clean up the area by smoothing foundation or pressed powder around the outer edges of the lips. Cover the mouth completely with a neutral pencil, and dab on a thin layer of lipstick, concentrating color on the center of the mouth (avoid the corners and edges). It defies logic, but the more lipstick you put on, the more likely it is to migrate. And skip gloss altogether — it will lubricate your carefully applied color and send it running.

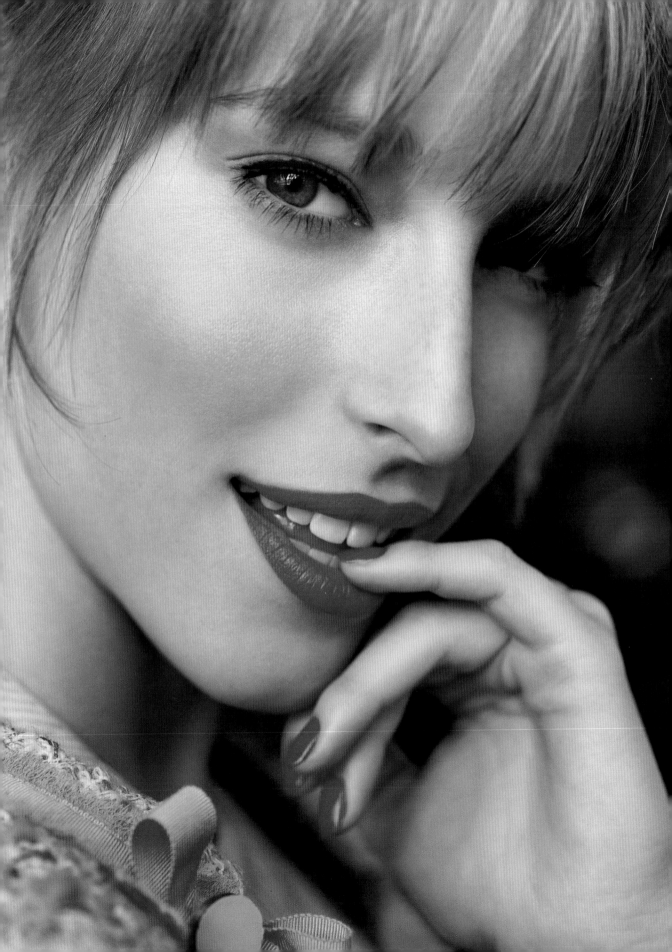

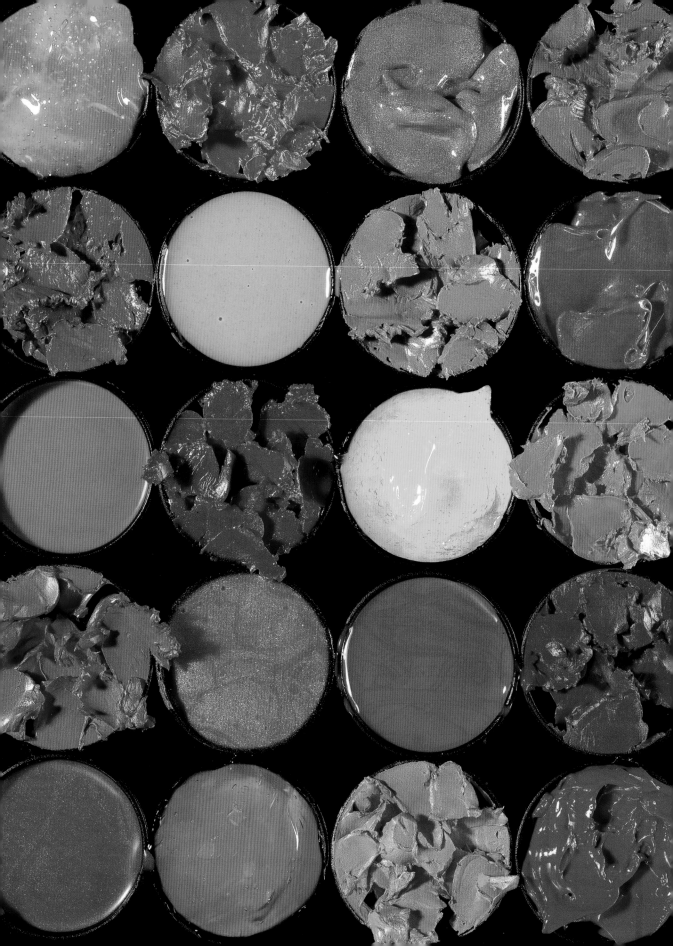

We've learned how to pick shades, and it doesn't involve buying dozens of lipsticks, only to realize they're all totally wrong.

We've hated so many shades that looked good in the store; once we got them home, we might as well have been wearing that green "mood lipstick" from the '80s. Here's how to pick a real winner.

IF YOUR SKIN IS FAIR, look for true pinks, nudes in slightly apricot shades, and dark berry colors. Stay away from anything brown, which will wash you out — unless you have pale skin smattered with freckles. In that case, pink-bronze hybrids look very pretty.

MEDIUM COMPLEXIONS CAN HANDLE A LITTLE MORE DEPTH. Instead of pink, try a stronger rose shade. Nudes can verge on peach, and when you go deep, consider a reddish burgundy instead of a pure red.

OLIVE-TONED SKIN IS FLATTERED MOST BY shades that have some brown — anywhere from bronze to raisin. Steer clear of candy pinks (unless you're a stripper) or any formula with white or silver (they make olive skin look sallow).

DARK SKIN can go in one of two directions: toward brown or purple. Think caramel or walnut for day, and plum or wine for evening.

AND NOW AN A.P.B.: Your lipstick should work with your skin and hair color and your mood, not your outfit. Don't match your gloss to your sexy new coral top, your boyfriend's tan jacket, or the red cocktail napkins at your favorite Italian restaurant.

Guilty as Charged

We rarely go to the matte.

Every few years, makeup artists manage to convince us that matte lipstick is back. But when it comes to our own mouth, we secretly think, Not a chance. While matte lipsticks have changed dramatically from dry, thick pigments to thinner, more comfortable silicone formulas, we still don't use them on a daily basis. Instead, we've learned how to turn any lipstick into a matte lipstick for a day: Pick a rich shade, like burgundy, apply one thick layer of color, then place a one-ply tissue over the mouth and lightly dust it with translucent powder. The result is a smooth, suedelike finish that never turns to distressed leather.

Beauty Myth

The Myth: Not everyone can wear red lipstick.

THE TRUTH: Bobbi Brown once declared that there really is a red for everyone, and we believe her. The trick is in the undertones — not the color. Fire-engine red looks best on women with warm complexions (like olive skin); cooler tones (fair or ruddy skin) should stick to cherry red; and dark-skinned women can have their pick of any crimson. Even the brightest redhead doesn't have to forswear red lipstick — just look at Julianne Moore.

Nude, in makeup, means fully dressed.

Nude lipstick provides the ultimate contrast against dramatic lashes and shadow. It also, however, can make you look like a corpse. Tips on staying alive:

FINDING A FLATTERING NUDE is like searching for the perfect pair of jeans — it may take a dozen tries to get the right fit. To narrow your options, look in the mirror: Your lipstick should never be lighter than your skin.

AVOID SHADES WITH WHITE UNDERTONES — they're horrible on everyone. Instead, choose a golden or pink-tinged hue.

FOR THE SEXIEST RESULTS, we heed the advice of makeup artist Tom Pecheux: Skip the liner so the lipstick is a little transparent (and doesn't look like misplaced concealer).

ALWAYS FINISH WITH A LIBERAL DOSE OF GLOSS — matte nude lipstick is truly the kiss of death.

We have to tell you some things you might not want to hear about lip liner.

We like to think there's an art to what we do, but there's also some science involved. Having conducted a rigorous interview of all the makeup pros we know, we can now say it's official: Visible lip liner is the number one beauty crime in America.

DO NOT USE SAID LINER TO DRAW A LINE — no matter how counterintuitive that sounds. Makeup artists scribble over the entire mouth with pencil, since it serves as an anchor for lipstick.

REPEAT AFTER US: Liner should never, ever be darker than your lipstick. You only need one that matches the shade of your mouth.

REMEMBER THAT '80S TREND of lining just outside the lips to make your mouth look fuller? Please don't. Only press-on nails look less natural.

Trick of the Trade

To make your lips look fuller, makeup artists dot their shiniest gloss right in the center of the lower lip.

Beauty Myth

The Myth: Lip plumpers can change the size of your pout.

THE TRUTH: Many of these serums and sticks contain ingredients like cinnamon, grapefruit, or hot peppers, which irritate the lips, causing them to swell slightly and feel briefly numb. Other formulas are packed with potent moisturizers, which hold water in the skin, making it a bit plumper. But any lip balm will do that. And to be honest, we've never found either variety to plump our pout in the least.

Gloss *can* last for more than six minutes.

Lip gloss is sort of like microwave popcorn — weightless, easy, and totally irresistible. Too bad it usually stays in place for about as long as it takes to polish off a bowl of Orville Redenbacher's. We've learned a few tricks for making it last.

PICK THE RIGHT GLOSS by looking for a few simple code words. Names that sound hard or thick ("lip lacquer," "glass," "diamond") will likely have more color, be nearly opaque, and stay put longer; wet words like "juicy" or "slick" are signs of sheer, ephemeral colors.

BEFORE GLOSSING, fill in the lips completely with a pencil that matches your mouth. (Warm the point between your fingers for several seconds first to soften so it doesn't leave any obvious marks.) After that, the real secret is a swipe of waxy balm — something about the consistency of Chap Stick — which will create a smooth, water-resistant base beneath the gloss.

PUCKER YOUR LIPS AS IF GIVING A KISS, then spread a small dot of shine (working in thin layers gives the most control) from the middle of the mouth to its perimeter by lightly patting with a fingertip or wand. Avoid going all the way to the rim, where color can bleed and look sloppy. If you want more color, dab on one more thin layer of gloss.

COUNTER INTELLIGENCE:
How to get a department-store makeover

We hate to break it to you, but those nice people behind the makeup counter would actually like to sell you something. That said, many are also trained makeup artists who can help you try on a new look while they're computing their commission.

1. Plan ahead.
To avoid a long wait, visit the store an hour after it opens or 90 minutes before closing (just steer clear of lunch hour and weekends). It's also a good idea to give the makeup artist a head start by exfoliating the night before and coming in with a clean face.

2. Look around.
When picking a counter and an artist, listen to your gut. If you're drawn to a particular line, odds are it will complement your aesthetic. And seek out a counter person whose own makeup is well applied, even if it isn't what you'd choose for yourself — it's the skill that matters.

3. Speak up.
Shy people get the worst makeovers. Describe your job, your wardrobe, the makeup you already own, the looks you hate — all this will clue in the artist to what you want. Then watch the entire application process. Tell her if you hate the catlike eyeliner she's applying, ask plenty of questions, and request a cheat sheet for the finished look. The "ta-da" moment may be fun, but it won't teach you much (and can be a very alarming surprise).

4. Know your rights — and obligations.
Unless a makeup artist tells you beforehand that there's a minimum purchase requirement (usually around $35 for an hour-long lesson), you are under no obligation to buy — but be prepared for an awkward moment and a nasty stare if you don't. For a makeup application before a party, it's customary to buy at least what you'd use for touch-ups (lipstick, gloss, and pressed powder).

5. Know when to walk away.
If a counter person launches into a hard sell, or you absolutely despise your result, don't capitulate. To escape, just use the words every clerk understands: "I'm going to walk around and look at the makeup in different lighting." Then bolt for the nearest bathroom sink.

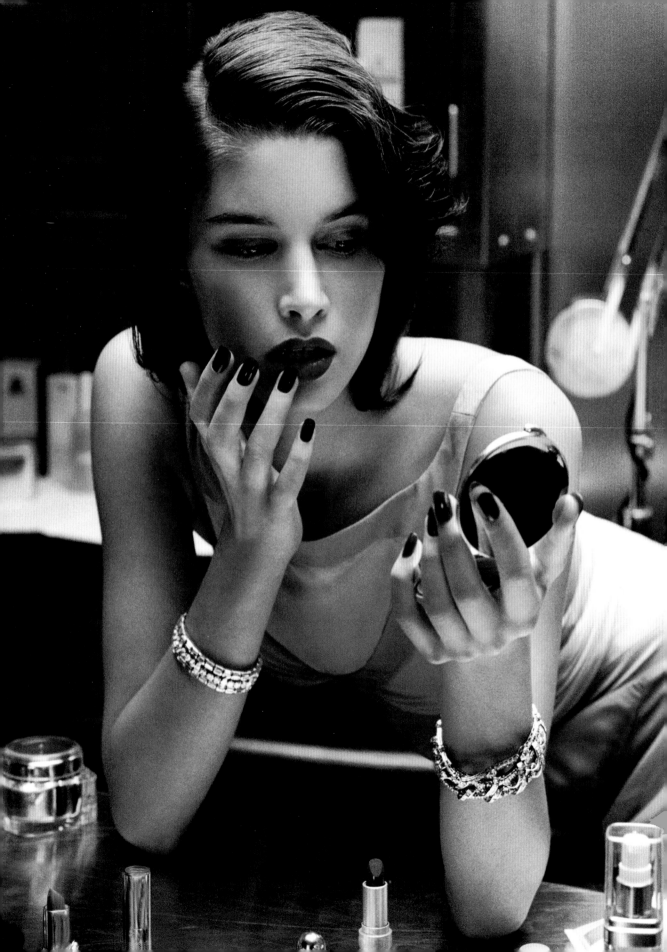

Dark colors are sexy and dramatic — and require a few extra tricks.

If sheer lip gloss is makeup's good girl, full-on dark lipstick is its moody older sister — sophisticated, sexy . . . and a little dangerous. While the right application and color produce instant femme fatale, one wrong step can be fatal (in beauty terms).

WHEN CHOOSING A BOLD COLOR, follow the makeup artists' rules: deep berry on fair skin, reddish burgundy on medium skin, brownish wine on olive skin, and deep purple on dark skin.

MOST PROS SKIP LIP LINER with dark shades because it can make the mouth look too harsh. Instead, they paint on color with a brush, starting at the center of the lips, and blend outward in short strokes. Work in thin layers until you have the intensity you want. Don't worry if the color isn't perfect around the edges — a lived-in look is more flattering (and younger).

IF YOUR LIPSTICK TENDS TO BLEED, fortify it first by running a brush or Q-tip dipped in translucent loose powder on the skin around your mouth *before* applying color. You can also replace lip balm with an anti-feathering gel or cream before you begin.

Trick of the Trade

To keep bold lipstick from smearing all over your teeth, try a trick we learned from makeup artist Mary Greenwell: After application, stick one finger in your mouth, and drag it out. This will remove just the color that's inside your lips.

BEAUTY SCHOOL
Long-Wearing Lipstick 101

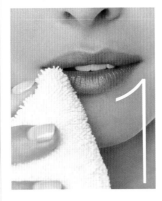

POLISH AND SEAL

Lipstick adheres best to a smooth surface. Once every two weeks, gently exfoliate lips with a soft toothbrush or a damp washcloth. (Skip this step if you are prone to cold sores.) Follow with a smear of balm — a waxy one will cement color.

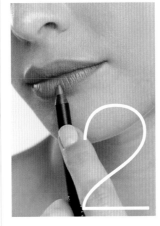

LINE AND FILL

A basecoat of liner helps lipstick endure. Steady your hand by resting an elbow on the bathroom counter. Then trace the vermilion border — the almost invisible line just at the edge of the colored part of the lips — with a liner that matches your mouth. Fill in lips completely with the side of the pencil, rather than the point, for a more even application of color.

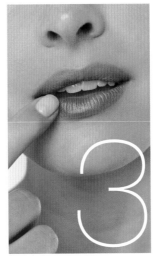

APPLY AND BLOT

For precision, apply a thin layer of color with a lip brush from the mouth's center, blending outward. Do not paint the corners. If you don't have a brush, dab the color from the tube. Blot with a tissue, then apply another layer of color. For extra strength, place a one-ply tissue over your mouth, dust with loose powder, remove the tissue, and add one more layer of lipstick.

The 10 Commandments

1

Color clings better to a smooth surface, so exfoliate lips once a week.

2

Lip liner should never, ever be visible.

3

A base layer of waxy balm can keep gloss from going MIA.

4

Your lipstick should coordinate with your skin color, not your outfit.

5

The most natural-looking lipstick is close to your own lip color, just glossier and slightly deeper.

6

Nude lipstick looks deadly unless it's topped with gloss or balm.

7

There truly is a red for everyone.

8

If you are going to wear dark lipstick, be prepared to touch it up.

9

Major lipstick calls for minimal eye makeup.

10

Combine a rosy pink lipstick with a dab of gloss at the center of the lower lip to make the mouth look bigger.

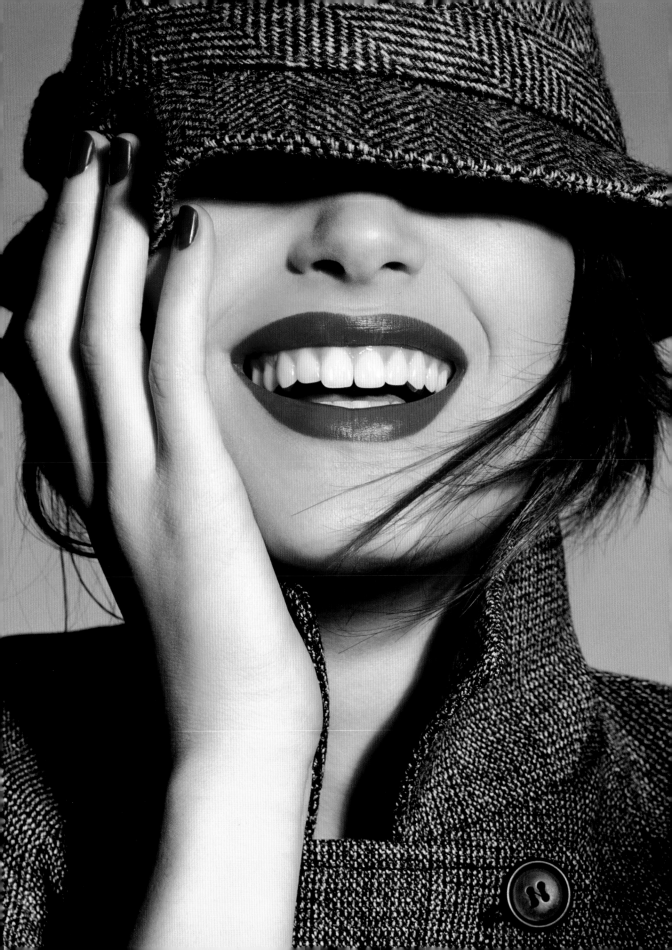

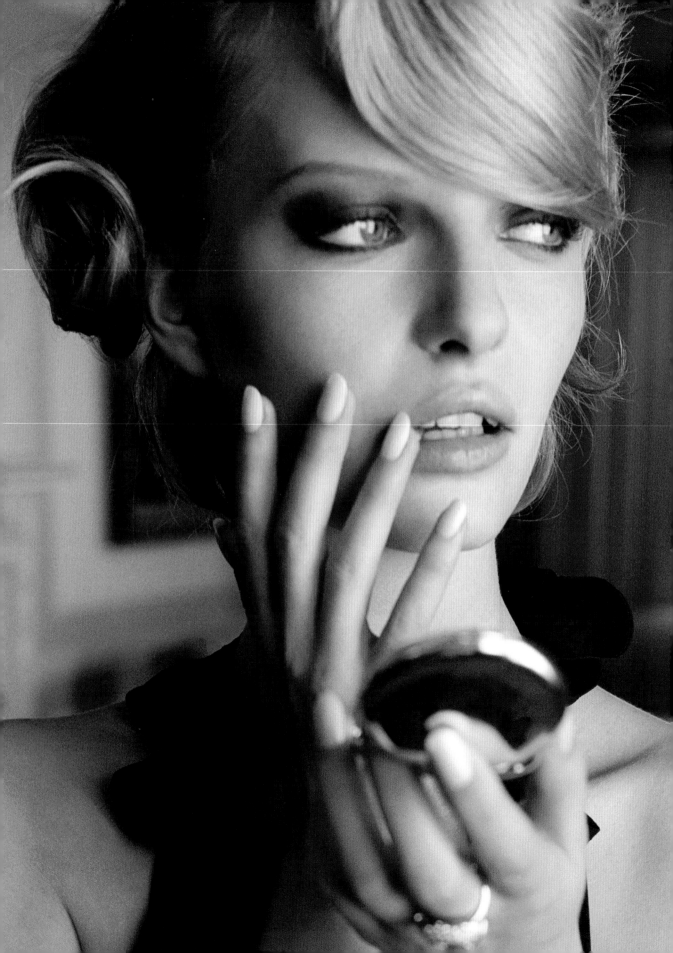

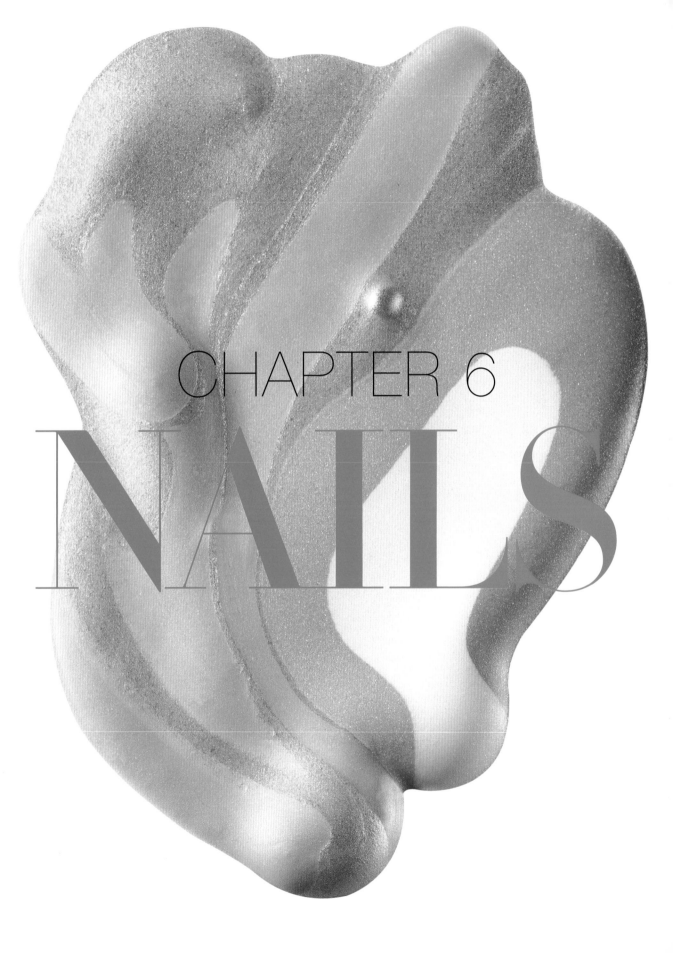

CHAPTER 6
NAILS

As I write this, my correspondence is tardy, my bedside table is buckling under a stack of unread books, and my spice rack is unalphabetized. My handwriting is so crabbed that I've been told I should have been a doctor. But my toes are perfect. Each one is pared and neatly polished — ten glossy little lozenges that no one sees. I know they're there, my order in chaos.

I had my first pedicure at the advanced age of 25. Now, at my neighborhood salon, eight-year-olds in braids have standing appointments and know exactly how much to tip and how long to hold their nails under the blowers before slipping on their shoes. Like them, I've become addicted. I'm not a massage person; facials leave me cold; scalp treatments, reflexology, and professional exfoliation are my idea of nothing to do. Pedicures are my weakness.

Sometimes beauty treatments are more than cosmetic. Their power as ritual eclipses any other benefit. With the ends of her hair neatly clipped, her roots carefully tinted, her eyebrows exactly arched, a woman feels that she is in command, in line, unfrayed. Of course, someone with this idea of order can become neurotic: I know one woman who, when her job was in jeopardy, would wait outside the locked door of her salon in the morning for a trim, a little color, anything to give her peace. When the ax finally fell, she looked like a million bucks.

Manolo Blahnik, the shoe designer, once told me that he can learn a lot about a woman just from a glimpse at her feet. "If the toes are fabulously groomed, that person is a perfectionist," he said. "Her mind is tidy and her house is in order." I'm sorry, Manolo. My toes are the beauty equivalent of false advertising. My mind may be messy, my house cluttered, but at least my feet are perfect.

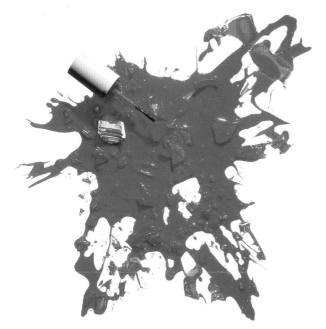

GETTING THIS SAME SHAPE at the salon is a little more complicated. (Seriously, just ask for a squoval, and see what happens.) Instead, try this little trick we've learned over the years: When the manicurist asks, "Square or round?" answer, "Square." Then, when she's filed the first nail, pipe up with, "Ooh, can you make it a little rounder?" and stop her when she hits the right shape.

A QUICK NOTE ABOUT LENGTH. We never grow our nails more than an eighth to a quarter inch past the tips of our fingers. Short nails look clean and stylish and prevent any visions of dragons.

There really is one nail shape that suits everyone.

We have a hard time keeping a straight face when we say it out loud, but top manicurists agree: The most flattering shape for nails is something called the "squoval," or squared-off oval.

IF YOU ARE DOING YOUR OWN NAILS, there's an easy way to know when you have the right contour: The tips should match the curve of your nail base. To get it, clip nails straight across, then round off the corners with an emery board. It's best to work from the outside toward the middle in one direction, not sawing back and forth (which gives you less control and can even cause splitting).

Trick of the Trade

If you are a nail biter, consider this trick from Ji Baek, owner of the New York City and Los Angeles Rescue Beauty Lounges: Anyone can stop if she commits to weekly manicures for 12 weeks. Not only is it a lot tougher to gnaw at a nicely filed and polished set of tips, but you'll also stop and think of all the money invested. Be warned that many women backslide around week three — persevere, and attractive nails can be yours.

Beauty Myth

The Myth: Eating Jell-O will give you strong nails.

THE TRUTH: Yes, gelatin contains protein, and protein contributes to healthy nails. But remember, you're eating it, not injecting it. And unless you suffer from a severe protein deficiency — something that's rare in the United States — consuming even a gallon of Jell-O every day wouldn't make a difference.

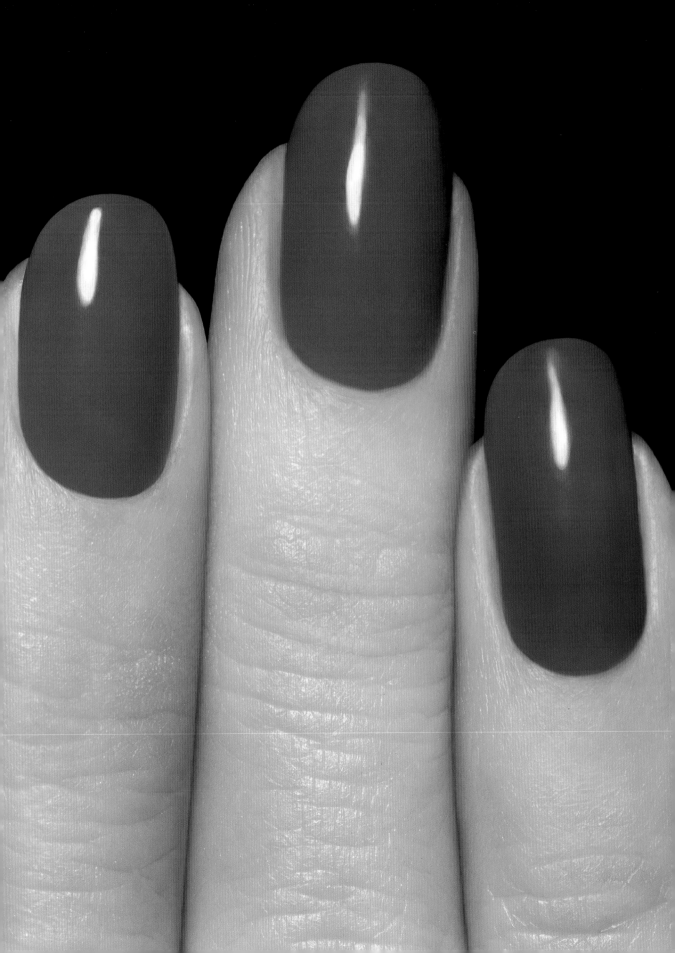

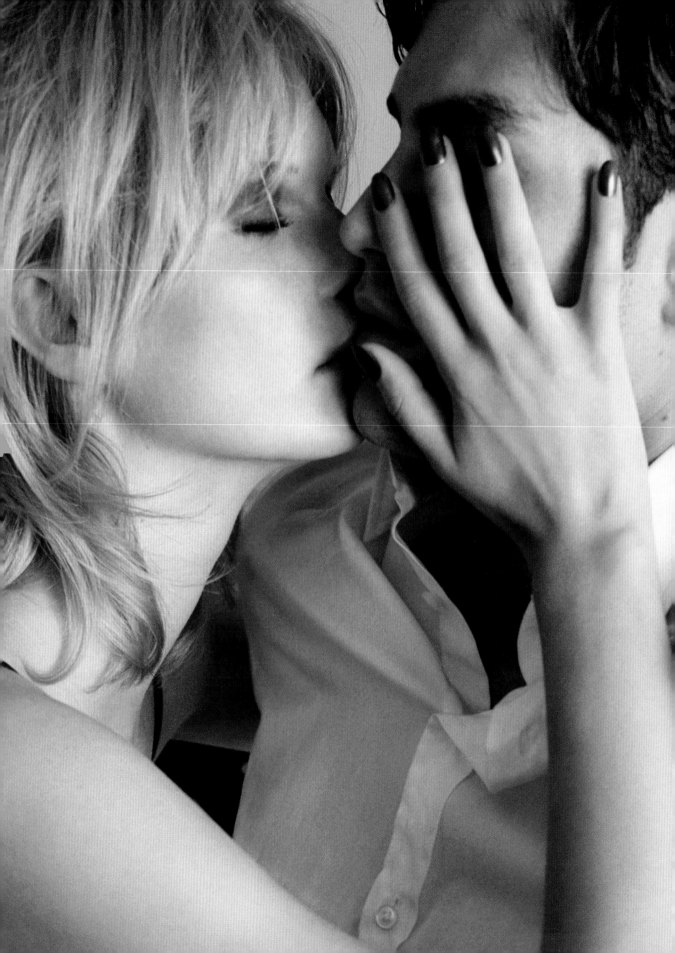

We're women of extremes.

We've learned that's it's hard to go wrong at the far ends of the nail-polish spectrum — pale pinks and beiges always look sweet and pretty, and dark, vampy reds scream sex. It's in the murky middle of actual colors and shimmer and French manicures that things get complicated (read: tacky).

WHEN WE WANT TO LOOK DRAMATIC, we go dark. For pale skin, this means fire-engine red or wine; for medium skin, bloodred or burgundy; for dark skin, garnet or eggplant.

GOING NUDE ON YOUR NAILS is far easier than, say, going nude on the Riviera. Sheer nude polish is the most forgiving if you're in a hurry, but if your nails are stained, discolored, or ridged, a more opaque shade with a golden or pink tinge is better. Just make sure the color doesn't contain too much white — that doesn't look natural on anyone.

METALLICS AREN'T AS SCARY AS THEY SEEM. If you tend to favor silver jewelry over gold (or vice versa), you've already figured out what flatters you. If not, there's an easy test: Grab something yellow and something blue, and hold them against the inside of your wrist to see which is closest to the undertone of your skin. Gold polish is right for yellow-based complexions; silver is for blue-based. As for the shimmer, the smaller the particles, the better — actual glitter is a little too fourth grade.

WE HAVE TO ADMIT IT: We just aren't big fans of bright colors on fingers. Toes, of course, are another matter — especially in winter. A splash of pink or tangerine can be positively uplifting, and there's no better time to experiment and find out what shades suit you than the months when feet are hidden in shoes all day long.

Cheater's Guide

We don't like to think of ourselves as commitment-phobic, but 45 minutes in a pedicure chair followed by 30 minutes of drying time can sometimes make us feel like bolting. Here's what we do instead: A few hours before going to bed, we paint on basecoat, then two coats of colored polish, without bothering to keep within the lines. Then we add a layer of topcoat. During our morning shower, we just reach down and scrape any stray polish off with our fingernails. It actually is that simple.

Trick of the Trade

Our bodies may need work, but at least our nails are buff. To keep them looking pink and shiny for two weeks, clean nails of all water and cuticle cream, then buff away. Choose a tool with four surfaces (they're usually numbered, from roughest to smoothest). Buff lightly, stroking horizontally three times — once on each side, then once in the middle — with each surface until you get the shine you want.

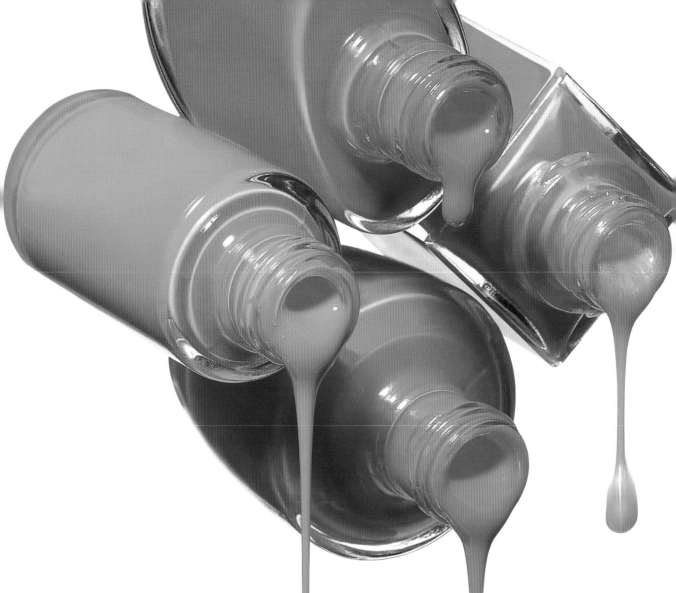

We've learned a thing or two from all those hours in the manicurist's chair.

It's not quite writing Bible verses on a grain of rice, but polish application is a painstaking process where small things make a big difference. Here are the finer points.

DON'T SHAKE THE POLISH BOTTLE as if you're mixing a martini — it can cause tiny air bubbles to form. Instead, roll it back and forth between your palms.

TO GET JUST THE RIGHT AMOUNT OF LACQUER on the brush, dip it into the bottle, and drag it up along the bottle's opening. The side of the brush with polish still on it will have enough to cover one nail.

THINK YOUR HANDS ARE TOO SHAKY to do your own manicures? Try resting your pinkie against an immovable object, like the bathroom sink, while painting. Your little finger isn't doing anything else, and an anchor can save the day.

HERE COMES THE HARD PART: You need to allow far, far more time for drying than you'd probably like. It takes 10 minutes for polish to set, and 30 to 45 (depending on the polish and number of coats) before you should even think about using your hands for anything other than dramatic gestures. Nails will still be soft enough to scuff for up to three hours.

Trick of the Trade

If you get a deep, dark, or bright paint job, consider buying a bottle of the polish to take home — these shades chip more often and more noticeably.

Manicure 101

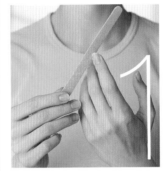

SHAPE
First, remove polish from nails. Cut straight across with clippers so nails extend no more than an eighth to a quarter inch beyond the fingertips. Then, stroke an emery board in one direction, from each side into the center, to round off the corners.

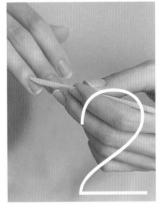

SOFTEN
Rub a generous amount of oil or moisturizer into the cuticles. Soak hands in a bowl of warm water with a splash of olive oil or milk — not soap, which can be drying. After three minutes, blot water from hands, and gently push back cuticles with an orange stick, a stone cuticle pusher, or even a damp washcloth. Wipe oils from nails with polish remover.

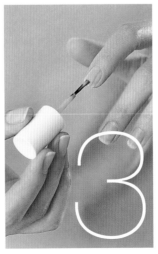

POLISH
Brush basecoat on the center of the nail from base to tip in one even stroke. Repeat on either side of the center stripe. Wipe the polish brush against the edge of the bottle, and placing it an eighth inch from the cuticle, paint on color in three quick stripes. Redip for each nail, and allow coat to dry at least two minutes before applying a second layer. Seal polish with topcoat. Correct mistakes with a cotton-wrapped orange stick dipped in remover.

Diamonds may be a girl's best friend, but topcoat is a close second.

Chipped polish is like visible panty lines. Both are a little trashy looking and entirely avoidable. Fortunately, a little prevention goes a long way when it comes to peeling, scuffing, smudging, and chipping.

ALWAYS START BY SWIPING NAILS with remover to rid them of oil and moisture, even if you aren't wearing polish. The new polish will adhere better to a totally dry surface. If your nails have ridges (which can be especially noticeable when covered in metallic polish), lightly sand them down with a buffing block. Just stop when the surface looks matte — polish won't stick as well if the nail is shiny.

IF YOU HAVE TIME, apply two layers of basecoat. Not only will it make colored polish stick better, but it also protects nails from discoloring.

CONTRARY TO POPULAR BELIEF, topcoat is not a one-shot deal. Manicurists recommend reapplying a thin coat every other day — even daily in the summertime, when UV rays can give polish a nasty yellow tinge.

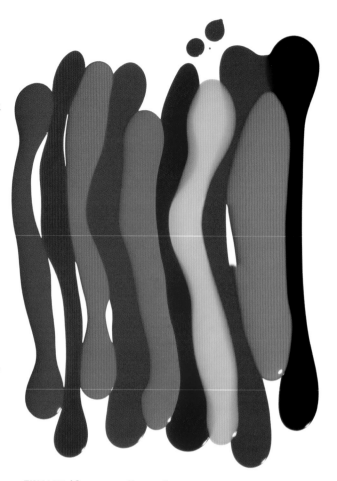

FINALLY, if you really, truly want to prevent chipping, we've got two words for you: rubber gloves. Your nails are like sponges — every time you splash around in soapy water or take a shine to Windex, they absorb the chemicals and dry out, loosening the polish from the nail and weakening the nail itself.

Beauty 911

Your home manicure was going just fine — until you got fuzz on the wet polish.

With all those cotton balls lying around, it's bound to happen. Use your cuticle nippers or a pair of tweezers to pull out the lint, being careful not to touch the nail. If the polish is marred, moisten the pad of your finger with polish remover, and tap it lightly on the divot to smooth it. Cover with topcoat.

Slip into a pair anytime you feel strangely compelled to do housework.

We don't go running to the salon for every little chip and scratch.

So you took every precaution and still have a ding on your ring finger. Chips happen — but that doesn't mean you have to start over.

A MANICURIST ONCE TOLD US everyone should have a couple of buffing disks in their kit. When you notice a chip, buff the edges with one of those round, gentle disks. It doesn't need to be absolutely perfect, but the smoother the edges, the less noticeable the fix is going to be.

FILL IN THE CHIP by putting just a dot of polish on the brush, then carefully dab the color into the bare area. Let the nail dry for a minute or two, then sweep one coat of the same color polish over the entire nail.

IF ALL ELSE FAILS, admit defeat, and remove your nail polish. Bare nails look cleaner than chips any day.

Trick of the Trade

A lesson we've learned the hard way: If you nick your nail reaching for your wallet, stop and ask the manicurist for a professional fix. After all the time you've invested, what's another three minutes? And there's no reason to feel like an ass — she does this *all the time.*

CRASH COURSE

Salvaging a Torn Nail

Like a tiny hole in a sweater, a torn nail can be ignored — until it unravels your entire manicure. These tricks will save you a trip to the salon.

1 First, find out what you're up against. Spread the offending hand as wide as you can, and carefully remove the polish from the broken nail.

2 If the split is above the fingertip — and you are prepared to file down the other nails — go ahead and clip the offender at the point of the break. To keep the fissure from growing, be sure to trim enough so that no trace of the split remains.

3 If the break travels below the fleshy part of the fingertip, or you can't bear to chop off your other nails, go ahead and seal it. Take a tea bag, tear it open, and rip off a tiny scrap of the gauzy paper (a jagged edge actually blends more easily into the nail). Dab the crack in the nail with Krazy Glue, and drop the paper on top. Let it dry for five minutes, apply one more coat of glue, and wait five more. Smooth the patch with a fine-textured nail buffer, paint color on as usual, and commend yourself for being so crafty.

It's possible to paint your own toes even if you aren't a yoga master.

We love any excuse to recline in that vibrating salon chair and read trashy tabloids. But sometimes we have to take our pedicures into our own hands.

PREP TOENAILS — clipping, filing, and smoothing — as you would fingernails. To minimize contortions while polishing, and expletives shouted when the color smears all over the place, sit on a chair with your knees close to your chest. Hold the toe you're painting with your nonpolishing hand. If you're right handed, start polishing on your left foot, from pinkie to big toe (so your hand isn't hovering over freshly painted nails just begging to be smeared). Lefties should work from right to left.

STAINS CAN BE EXTRA STUBBORN on toenails — which is a problem when you've fallen in love with the latest sheer pink or nude. If discolorations can't be buffed away, conceal them by applying a light opaque polish as a first coat and then following with a matching sheer.

Pedicures aren't the only way to rub out rough skin.

Start with a clean slate by getting a professional pedicure (or even an appointment with the podiatrist, if calluses or ingrowns are a problem). After that, skin softening is merely a matter of maintenance.

IF YOU RUB A DOLLOP OF BODY SCRUB onto your heels during every single shower and follow with moisturizer once you get out, you shouldn't have to do anything else to keep your feet soft.

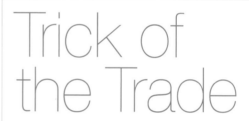

Trick of the Trade

Keep nail polish in the refrigerator — the cold preserves the consistency and keeps it from separating.

Beauty Myth

The Myth: Fast-drying topcoats are the best way to preserve your manicure.

THE TRUTH: If you're in a hurry, fast-drying formulas can be the way to go — as long as you understand that they are fast to chip, too. (The same goes for quick-dry polish.) Follow it up the next day with a layer of regular topcoat to ensure that your manicure isn't undone before the salon's charge is recorded on your credit card.

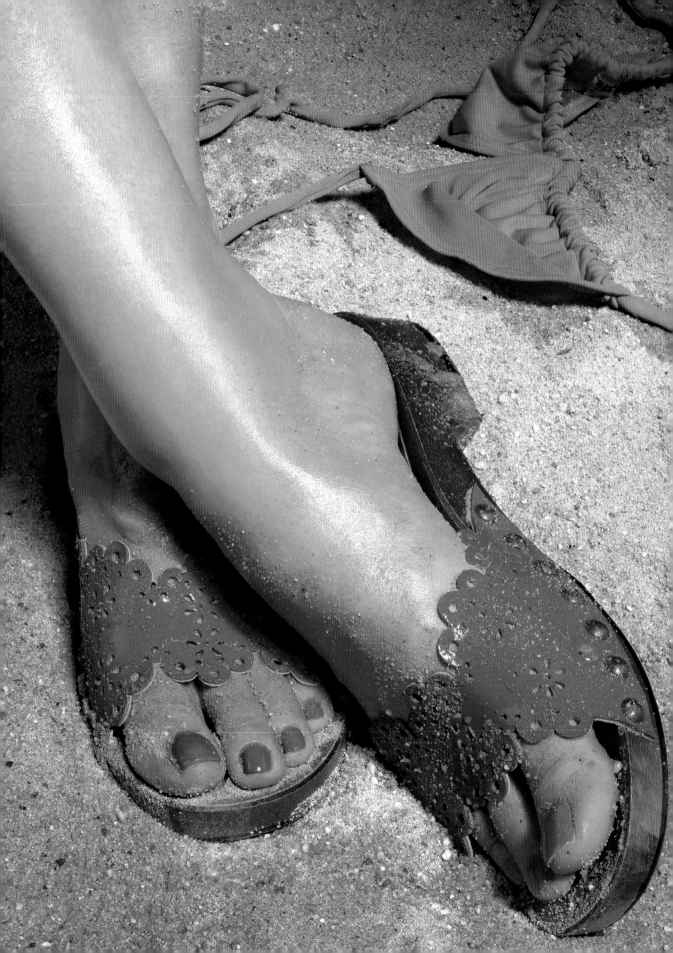

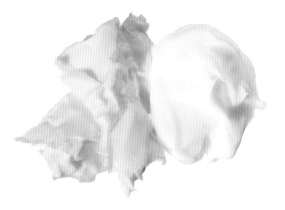

IF YOU ARE LESS THAN DILIGENT with the scrub or need a little extra ammunition, consider a foot file or rasp. (Manicurists prefer them over pumice stones, which can remove too much skin if you aren't careful.) Run it over tough spots in one direction after bathing, when skin is thoroughly dried, and follow with lotion. Any tube will do; special foot formulas tend to contain ingredients that break down dead skin cells, like urea or glycolic acid, but they're also too sticky for some.

OUR LITTLE PIGGIES may not be insured for millions, but we still employ a trick we learned years ago from a professional foot model. Once a week, slather feet in diaper-rash ointment (seriously), and slip them into a thin plastic bag — the kind you put lettuce in at the supermarket — before putting on a pair of socks and shuffling off to bed. You'll wake up to toes that are as soft as a baby's bottom. (You can also use body lotion or Vaseline, but where's the fun in that?)

All good things must come to an end.

OK, so removing nail polish isn't exactly rocket science. That doesn't mean we don't have opinions about it.

WHILE ACETONE-BASED REMOVERS ARE DRYING, nothing works better when it comes to banishing really dark polish. Just don't use them too often — more than once every two weeks can indeed be damaging to nails.

EVEN BASECOAT CAN'T TOTALLY INSULATE NAILS from polish pigment. If your nails are yellowed, try soaking them in a solution of four parts water to one part hydrogen peroxide (not bleach, which is too harsh) for ten minutes between manicures.

IF YOU ARE STRANDED WITHOUT REMOVER and feeling twitchy, resist the temptation to peel off your polish. We've done it, we've seen the flaking and damage it causes, and we'll never do it again.

Guilty as Charged

We can't resist a cuticle snip.

We've warned against it in the pages of *Allure* and recoiled in horror from tales of gruesome infections. But we are weak, *weak,* when the manicurist sweetly chirps, "You want me to cut your cuticles?" The truth is, the cuticle's sole purpose is to repel bacteria, viruses, fungi, and water from the nails — and cutting it only makes it more ragged in the future. The real solution lies in daily maintenance (which isn't as bad as it sounds). When you get out of the shower, take 20 seconds to push the cuticles back with the rigid corner of a damp towel. And since the other culprit behind raggedy flecks of skin is dryness, rub salve onto the cuticles daily. It doesn't have to be a cuticle oil; over the years, top manicurists have confessed to using olive oil, lip balm, and eye cream — anything that keeps skin hydrated will do.

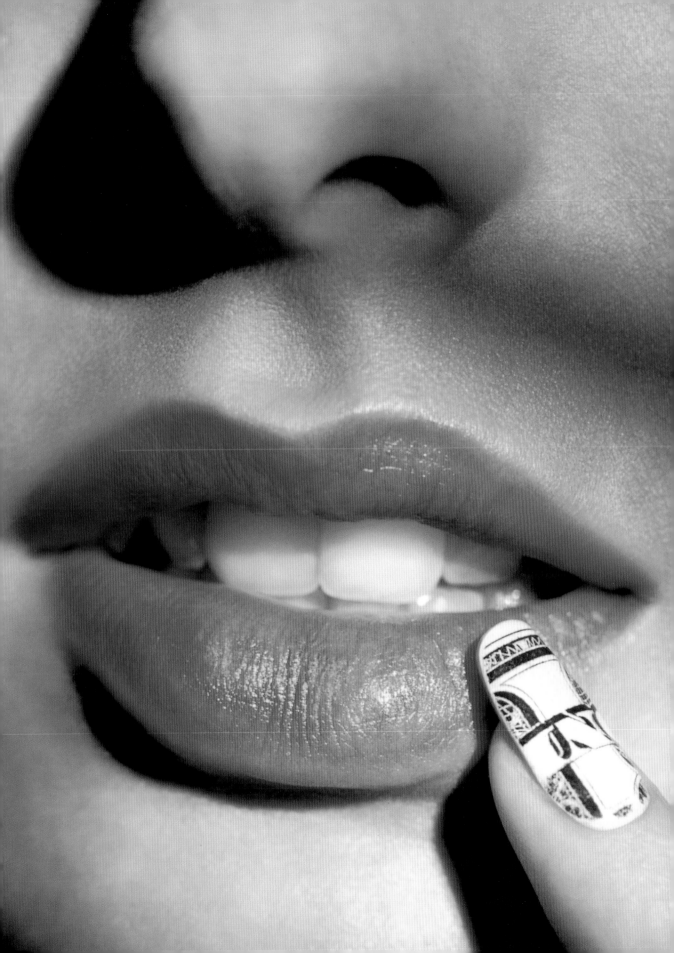

The 10 Commandments

1
Squared-off oval nails
are the most flattering shape
on nearly everyone.

2
The best length is an eighth to a
quarter inch beyond the fingertip.

3
Don't let anyone cut your
cuticles. Push them back
daily instead.

4
Basecoat creates a smooth
surface and prevents
discoloration: Use it.

5
The best nail colors are
either light and natural or
dark and vampy.

6
Paint three thin stripes
of polish, not one big glob,
on each nail.

7
If you don't want
smudges, allow 30 minutes
for nails to dry.

8
Reapply topcoat every
other day to keep nail
polish from chipping.

9
When your nail polish turns
yellow or chips, admit defeat,
and remove it all.

10
Get a pedicure at least
once a month.

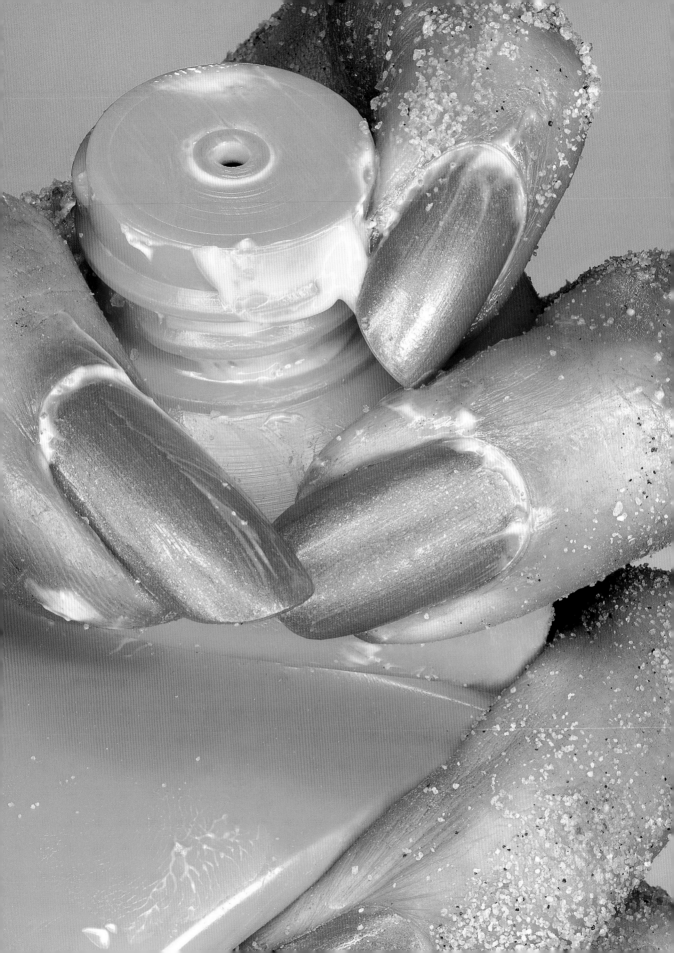

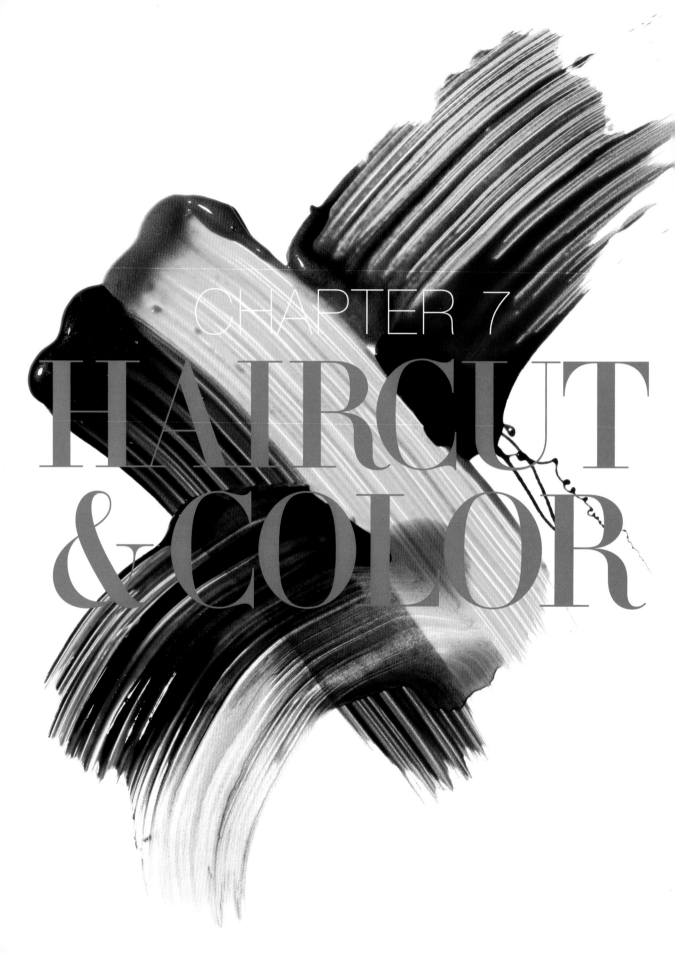

CHAPTER 7

HAIRCUT & COLOR

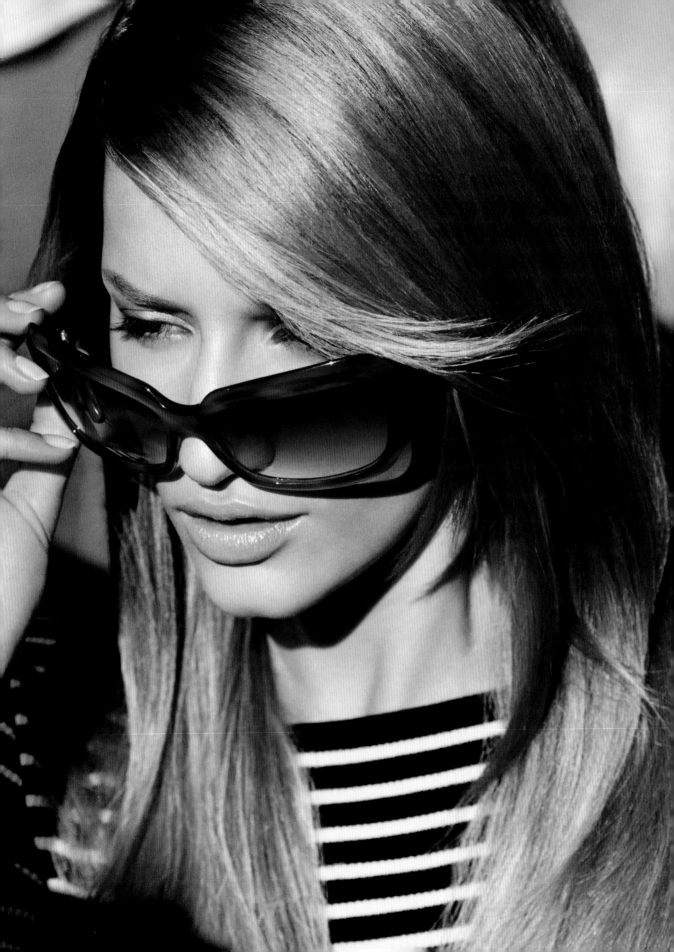

Like many women, I feel slightly cheated in the hair department. Where my brothers and sons have thick blond mops that practically need a garden rake to tame, my hair is scrawny, straight, and lank; it looks painted on my scalp. Despite heroic efforts from the finest stylists, my hair seemed destined for blandness. Long ago, I resigned myself to a blunt, shoulder-length cut, the kind that almost begs for a velvet headband and a country-club membership. I wore it parted slightly to one side, blow-dried it with my head flipped over, and pushed it behind my ears. That's where it remained, day after day after day.

When I took my usual seat at my longtime stylist Garren's salon one spring day, we both decided out of the blue that it was time for a change. I didn't discuss this in advance with my husband or friends, didn't take a poll or try on a short wig. I just gave Garren the nod, and he raised his scissors to the middle of my ear. Off went four inches of security. Scissors flashed, hair drifted to the floor, and I felt slightly dizzy. When he cleaned off my neck and stepped back, Garren seemed to have brushed away the cobwebs along with the length. I felt energized and new.

I've spent years analyzing the meaning of other women's haircuts, believing a big change precipitates other, more profound alterations. A woman cuts her hair or dyes it red and then quits her job, has an affair, moves to Greece, becomes a vegan, enters rehab. In my case, to paraphrase Sigmund Freud, the haircut was just a haircut.

But the reactions to the haircut were not entirely positive. One night, I ran into a cosmetics executive in the ballroom of the Waldorf-Astoria. He looked at me, winced, and said, "You cut your hair," with such disapproval that you'd think I'd sprouted horns as well. "I like it better long. This makes you look" — he paused, searching for the right word — *"older."*

"Well, thanks," I said in disbelief. "I've always wanted to look . . . older." I was tempted to add that his suit made him look . . . fatter. But that would have been . . . ruder.

There's no question I'd outgrown my girls'-school haircut; I *am* older. And I don't want to be one of those women who clings pathetically to a hairstyle or lip color long past its expiration date. Mr. Executive is entitled to his opinion. But I have to disagree. What I like about my new haircut is that it feels spirited and unpredictable, which is another way of saying "younger."

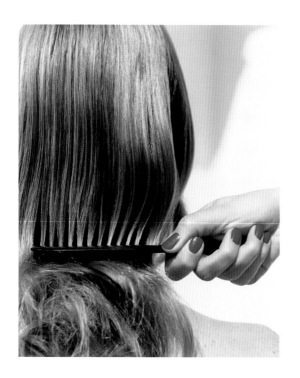

We've found the perfect cut for every hair type.

We once polled our readers about their hair, and a whopping 92 percent of them had major complaints ranging from frizz to flatness. (The other 8 percent, we suspect, are bald.) And while you might guess that hair salvation is found in the right products, the real road to enlightenment begins at the salon.

IF YOUR MAIN FOE IS LIMPNESS, length matters. Some stylists say the best cut is no longer than the shoulders; others advise stopping just below the chin. Whatever looks best on you, be sure to ask for blunt ends (they encourage thickness) and long, face-framing layers, not short, choppy ones, which may seem to add volume at first, but the illusion doesn't last. Consider eyebrow-skimming bangs: They can also help create the impression of fullness.

WOMEN WITH NATURALLY WAVY HAIR (the lucky things) should stay away from overly blunt cuts, which create a bushy mess at any length. The solution is jagged ends and plenty of layers. Ones placed at cheekbone level keep waves from overwhelming your face.

TRULY CURLY HAIR NEEDS SOME LENGTH to weigh it down; cut it too short, and that's when the poodle references begin. Ask for long layers, so the front pieces hit the top lip and then gradually angle back to create a shoulder-grazing shag.

STRAIGHT, THICK HAIR is especially vulnerable to frizz. Taming it begins with scrupulously neat ends, which means absolutely no razoring or serrated cutting (sliding the scissors down the hair shaft). Instead, ask for layers cut with something called a graduated point, a technique that involves little diagonal cuts. It will make the hair look softer and allows the layers to flow into each other.

Beauty Myth

The Myth: Split ends can be eliminated by braiding hair, then snipping off any visible frays.

THE TRUTH: Bad idea. You'll probably just end up with a ragged line. Instead, suck it up, and book yourself an appointment for a trim.

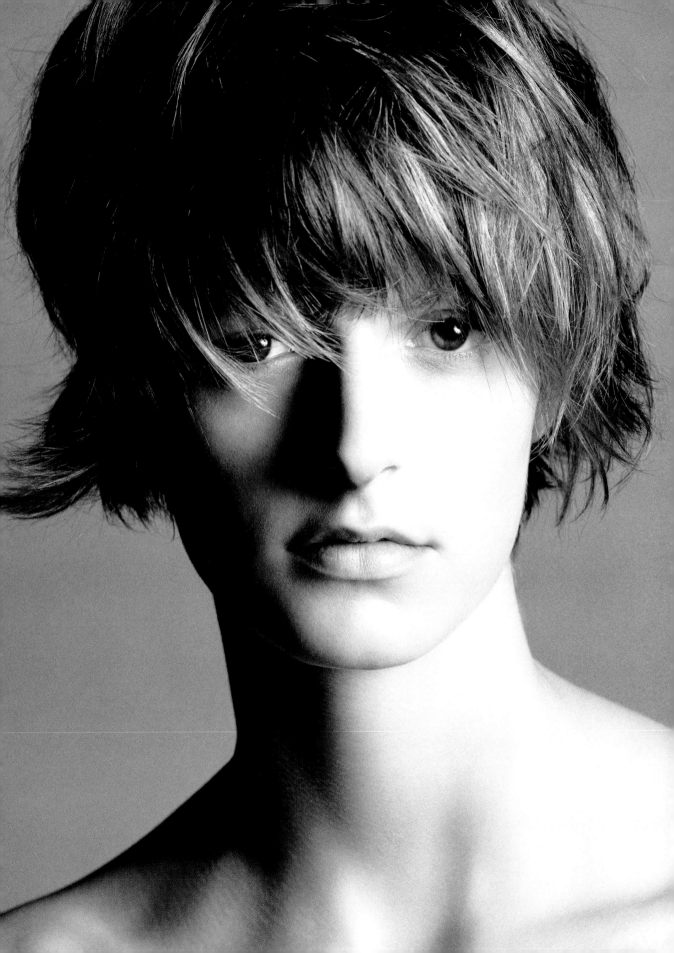

We know how to speak a stylist's native language.

In the drama-filled atmosphere of the salon, the best way to communicate with a stylist is usually the most straightforward.

BE SUCCINCT ABOUT WHAT YOU WANT, then volley back by saying, "So what do you think? Is this possible for my hair?" It shows you respect the stylist's opinion and won't irrationally insist on the impossible dream. If you aren't sure how to describe your ideal haircut, feel free to bring a photo — he won't find it insulting in the least. Stylists are visual people, and pictures neatly eliminate the ambiguity of words.

AVOID TALKING IN TERMS OF INCHES. Measurements may seem scientific, but have you ever seen a ruler in a salon? If you have hair to your collarbone and want it cut above your shoulders, hold your hand to that exact point, and show the stylist.

DON'T BE AFRAID TO SPEAK UP. Rather than burying yourself in a magazine, watch as the stylist works. If your hair seems too long after the cut, for example, go ahead and say so. And if he asks you questions about your daily routine, don't give ideal-world answers. If you really aren't willing to blow-dry every day, say so.

KNOW THE CODE WORDS. "Beachy" means hair that's a little roughed up, generally with wavy layers and a windblown look (which may require thickening sprays to maintain on a daily basis). "Piecey" refers to ends that are separated and defined (usually with wax or pomade), often on a shag or shorter style. "Structure" means a sharp, geometric cut à la the Vidal Sassoon bob, versus "movement," which usually translates as plenty of layers.

Cheater's Guide

We preach the importance of a flawless, high-class cut as the foundation of all hair happiness . . . and then a credit card bill arrives with a whole extra digit attached, and we find ourselves sneaking into a tawdry local salon for a quickie. If you're going to cheat on your stylist, take a few simple precautions. Ask the new stylist simply to follow the lines of your original cut, just trimming off the ends (with scissors, never a razor) until you have a classic, shoulder-grazing cut with long layers throughout. Whatever you do, don't ask for a blunt cut — it's actually one of the most complicated, and you may end up with tufts sticking out in weird places.

Beauty Myth

The Myth: Hair will grow faster and thicker if it's cut frequently.

THE TRUTH: Each strand is a thread of dead protein, and it certainly doesn't have any kind of feedback mechanism that would let the root know what's going on at the end. Since the root is where growth takes place, extra trips to the salon won't make hair grow faster (although trims will help it look better and fuller than straggly frayed ends).

We've figured out how long is too long — and how short is too short.

Allure editors come in all shapes and sizes, but a suspiciously high percentage of us have shoulder-length hair. The reason isn't laziness or fear (honest), but the undeniable fact that a shoulder-length cut tends to be the most universally flattering. For the bold who want to go longer or shorter, a few guidelines.

THERE ARE ONLY A COUPLE of hard and fast reasons to deny yourself flowing hair. First is the shape of your face and your body. Collarbone-length hair can drag down a long face and overwhelm a narrow one; if you're short, long hair really can overpower your body. The other disqualifier is damage: If your hair is brittle, frizzy, or stringy, it's going to look worse in abundance. Age alone isn't a deal breaker, though — if you're over 40, just remember that hair tends to thin over time.

THE PRECISE LENGTH OF HAIR that flows down the back is a lot less important than what you do with the pieces falling down your front. Cut lip- and chin-grazing layers if you possess any of the following: a gorgeous jawline, a long face, and/or thick hair. And since no bell goes off when your hair has grown too long, consider our personal rule: Once it passes the breasts, it's spooky, not sexy.

STRAIGHT, VOLUMINOUS HAIR adapts best to a short cut. If you have curly or frizzy hair, beware — it'll likely morph into a ball, a box, or a pyramid.

WITH SHORT HAIR, you can end up too bubble-headed if you have a round face or a short neck; the very tall run the danger of suddenly resembling candidates for the WNBA. And if you aren't willing to do the work, forget it. Short cuts are anything but — they require more products and more commitment in trims every three to six weeks.

We have our own big bang theories.

When we were little, bangs were so simple: Either you had them, or you didn't. Now there seems to be an endless variety: side-swept layers; soft and choppy; a blunt, bold slash just above the brows. Figuring out which ones are right for you is mainly a matter of your facial features and hair texture.

LONG, THICK HAIR IS MADE FOR BANGS. In fact, without them, hair beyond your shoulders can seem like curtains hanging on the side of your head. If hair is wispier, make bangs look as thick as possible by cutting them so they're wide and start farther back on the head (though not so much so that the rest of the hair looks limp in comparison).

Trick of the Trade

Cutting off cherished long hair can be traumatic, so consider easing yourself in step-by-step. First, take a picture of yourself against a dark background, and use a Sharpie to black out your hair to the desired length to see how it might look. Then try wearing it back every day for a week: This will show you what your face really looks like, and you can decide if you're comfortable exposing it.

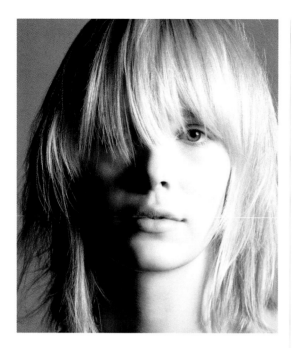

CRASH COURSE
Trimming Your Own Bangs

We bitched so much to our stylist about having to slog to the salon for bang trims that he finally taught us how to do it ourselves. Start by resisting the urge to wet hair — it's actually easier to see what you're doing when it's dry — and by using real haircutting scissors (they don't have to be pricey, just specifically designed for hair). Then divide bangs into three sections, grab the first one, pull it straight up in the air, and twist it like a unicorn's horn. Snip into the ends with the point of the scissors cutting diagonally a little at a time so that each strand is a slightly different length. Drop the section to see where it falls, then twist and cut some more if necessary. Pull up the next section, matching it to the length of the cut portion before snipping. And voilà — you just bought yourself a few more weeks.

BANGS DRAW ATTENTION TO THE NOSE, but that doesn't mean they're off limits to those of us with big honkers — witness Cher in her Sonny and . . . days. Just don't do it halfway in the form of wisps or side-swept bangs; the short, blunt version that stops just above the brows is more dramatic and flattering.

TO MAKE THE MOST OF A SMALL FOREHEAD, bangs should be as long as possible and start farther back on the head than usual. The reverse works, too: A large forehead can be hidden with bangs that are longer at the temples than at the middle.

A WARNING TO WOMEN with very curly hair or strong cowlicks: Bangs can be your worst nightmare. Unless they are heavy and long, or chemically straightened, they'll revert to their natural state at the first hint of humidity.

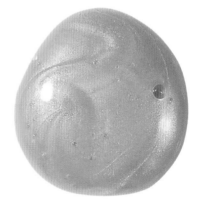

We've discovered the pros and cons of going blond . . .

No one will ever be able to determine definitively if blonds have more fun. But we're quite certain they have more disposable income and time on their hands, because going blond takes serious maintenance (just ask the 46 million American women who regularly lighten up). A few things to consider before you hit the bottle:

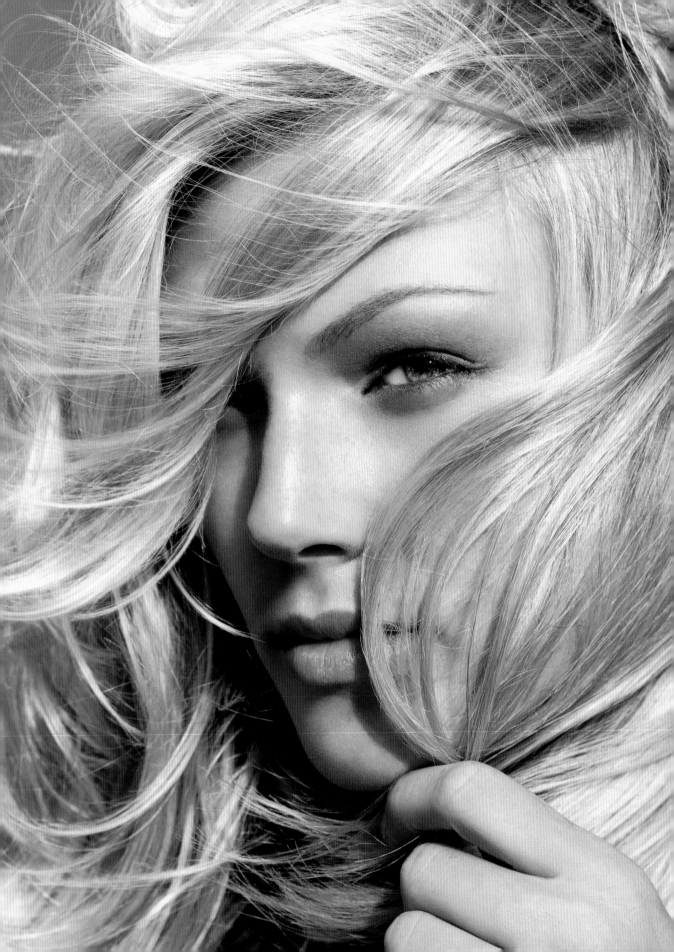

IF YOU HAVE OLIVE SKIN or have to go more than five shades lighter to get to blond, step away from the bleach. The best candidates are women who were blond when they were children, even if their hair has long since darkened.

CONSIDER YOUR SKIN TONE. Your hair and your skin should never be the same color. If you have sallow skin with yellow undertones, stay away from deep golds; if you have pinkish skin, avoid strawberry shades. A good colorist knows these things intuitively; in the drugstore, you're on your own, so don't go more than two shades in any direction, to minimize the potential for disaster.

WITH SHADES OF BLOND, more is more. Since multiple contrasting shades look more realistic than one monotone color, a single-process bleaching is unwise.

KNOW WHEN TO STOP. Sure signs of "blondrexia" are a constant need to add more makeup, visible roots in just a week or two, or serious breakage. When this happens, consult a pro.

DON'T FORGET YOUR BROWS. A good rule of thumb is that they should be tinted to match the darkest highlight (or the base color underneath, if you're doing overall lightening).

. . . and the pros and cons of going brown.

Anyone who's seen Elizabeth Taylor in her prime knows there's nothing inherently bland about brown — especially in Valrhona-chocolate-worthy combinations of cocoa, chestnut, and dark cherry.

IF YOU HAVE ESPECIALLY PALE SKIN, don't demand to go too dark — jet hair and light skin can be ghostly (and aging) on women over 30. The effect can usually be averted by adding warmer brown highlights around the face.

TAKE BABY STEPS. Experts recommend going no more than two shades darker the first time around. Sometimes a small change is the most flattering (and you can always go back for more if it's not).

THE TYPE OF DYE MATTERS. For darkening, top colorists like semipermanent formulas, which add a translucent shine to hair and don't contain damaging peroxide or ammonia. Permanent dye can make dark hair look like a wig.

REVEAL YOUR HAIR HISTORY. Dyed, permed, straightened, or otherwise processed hair is more porous, so it grabs color more easily than virgin strands. Always tell your colorist exactly

Beauty 911

A few too many laps in the pool have left your blond hair looking positively green.

Home remedies are remarkably effective on this particular problem. Colorist Negin Zand, who's responsible for Nicole Kidman's and Kate Hudson's blond locks, swears by rinsing tresses in V8. If that sounds like Sunday brunch gone bad, crush three aspirin into a couple of ounces of water, mix until it forms a paste, apply to hair, and wait five minutes before rinsing it out.

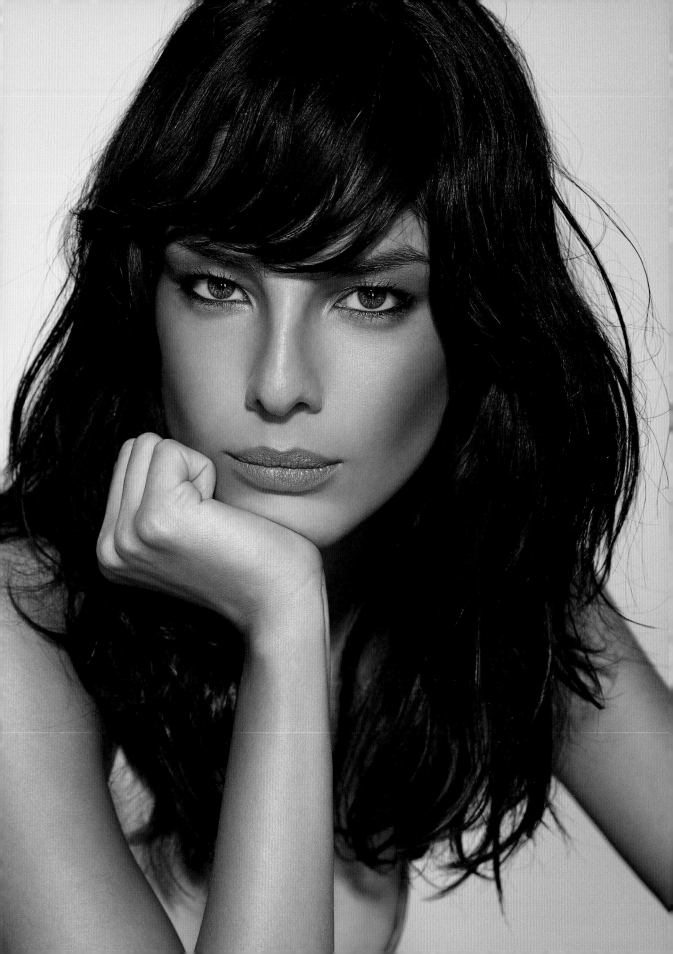

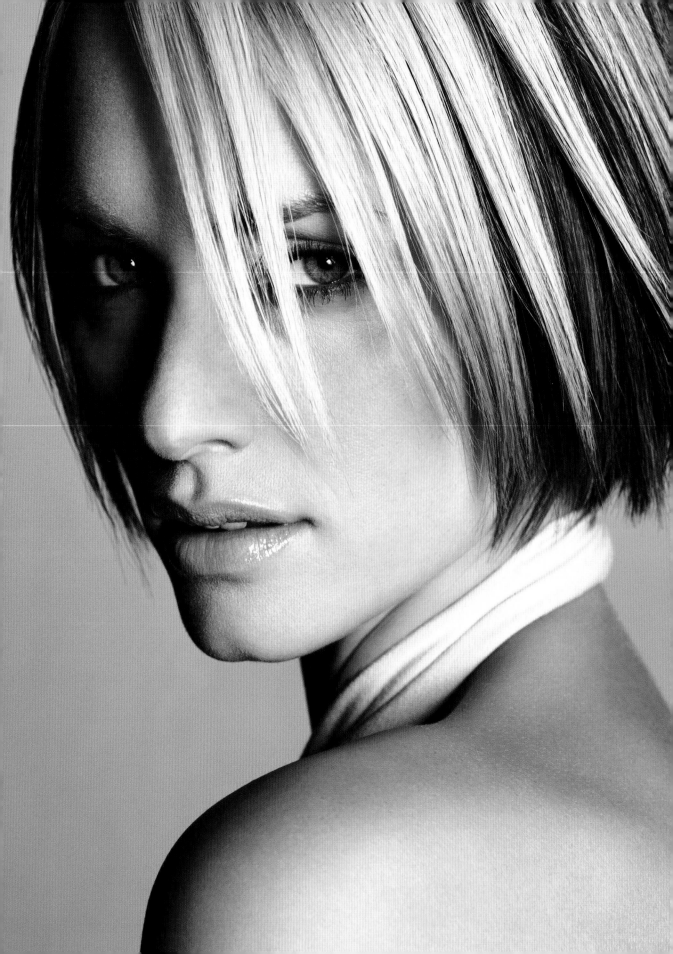

what you've done to your hair, as far back as you care to remember — even if you straightened it a year ago, you could end up with weirdly dark tips.

CONSIDER BRINGING PHOTOS. One person's mahogany is another's espresso, and for some reason this confusion seems more rampant with shades of brown than with blond.

We've finally figured out how to dye our hair over the bathroom sink.

As anyone who has ever paid $150 for a single-process dye job can attest, applying one shade of color isn't a terribly complicated matter. With do-it-yourself kits, it's not what you use, but how you use it. Go slowly, and keep changes to a minimum, and you can tell any lie you want about what salon you go to (not to mention save about $138).

HAIR THAT'S TOO LIGHT OR TOO DARK drains the color right out of your skin, so stay within two shades of your natural color when flying solo. And don't join the shockingly high percentage of dyers who don't bother to do a strand test before going full steam ahead, unless you want to find out what a full head of orange frizz looks like.

ON SECOND THOUGHT, don't fly solo — grab a friend (and a jar of Vaseline). The friend will help you reach the back of your head; the Vaseline, spread around your hairline, will keep your forehead from turning inky. And start the project when the hair-color company's help line is open (in other words, not at midnight on Sunday).

WATCH A PROFESSIONAL COLORIST AT WORK and you'll see that hair is lighter around the face — yet we tend to buy only one box of hair color.

Guilty as Charged

We're tardy for our color touch-ups.

Everyone has different dreams about what they'd do if they won the lottery. While it isn't high on our list, having the time and money to get our color touched up every two weeks would be on there somewhere. In the meantime, we've come up with a few sneaky strategies for hiding roots. For starters, wear hair in a wavier, less structured style that is less likely to show demarcations. Consider moving your part — either flipping it to the other side (if you don't have any cowlicks) or just making it jagged instead of straight. And don't try to hide behind a ponytail. That only makes roots more noticeable.

Trick of the Trade

Be proactive: If your highlights tend to fade to orange stripes, or your blond turns platinum white, tell your colorist. She will adjust the formula accordingly and know which products will help your particular color last.

Instead, buy two shades, and apply the ever so slightly lighter one sparingly around the face.

ONE NOTE ON THOSE BOXES: It's best to ignore the picture on the front. It's the color chart on the side that matches results to your natural hair color.

MOST AT-HOME USERS MAKE THE MISTAKE of frying or overdarkening their ends. Repeat dyers should slick a generous amount of conditioner on the ends and apply color only to the roots. Five minutes before color is ready to be rinsed, refresh the ends by working the dye over the conditioner. (It's enough time, we swear.)

HERE'S A TRICK WE LEARNED from celebrity colorist Louis Licari. If you've finished your application and the color is too tame, take another box of dye, and dilute it with equal parts shampoo. Lather, let it sit for five minutes, and rinse — you'll add just enough color and a lot of shine.

Bad haircuts or highlights aren't forever.

Maybe it was the slip of a stylist's scissors, or perhaps you're the one who said, "What the hell, I've always wanted to be a redhead." Assigning blame won't help matters over the next few weeks while your hair grows in. Here's what will:

IF THE PROBLEM IS HEAVY BANGS or choppy ends, go to another stylist who can at least soften and blend them. An overlayered cut can sometimes be brought back into proportion by taking a bit off the back. But once the problem is under control, the experts are unanimous: Stay away

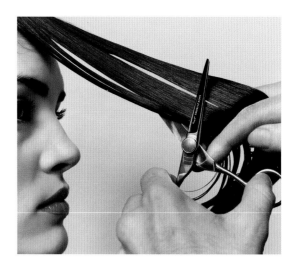

from the salon. Time heals all wounds, even to your pride.

WHILE YOU'RE WAITING out a bad cut, creative accessories can help. Stylist Serge Normant taught us to buy two or three thin strips of colored elastic from a sewing-supply store and then wear them twisted together as a headband. And unflattering short layers can be smoothed down and clipped close to the head with plain bobby pins (don't add insult to injury with ones adorned with butterflies or flowers, please). Women with straight hair who are phasing out longer layers can make them seem less choppy by creating a few waves with a large-barrel curling iron.

WHEN YOU GET SICK OF HIGHLIGHTS, it's tempting just to dye all your hair back to its natural color, but that rarely gives the desired effect. When dyes are applied to bleached hair, they can turn it ashy or greenish. Growing out your highlights gradually is better. Ask your stylist to add darker lowlights to your roots as they grow in. This will mute the contrast, and eventually the two will match. You can also use lowlights on the colored portions to make the highlights less pronounced.

What's Your Damage?

Deep conditioners and shine sprays can only go so far. Sometimes the best cure for wrecked strands is a rest.

THE PROBLEM: *Hair dries faster than it used to.* If medium-thick hair takes less than an hour to air-dry, it's in trouble. Avoid the blow-dryer and flatiron as often as possible.

THE PROBLEM: *Hair lacks elasticity.* Pluck one hair, and stretch it. If it doesn't spring back, hair could break if it's subjected to chemicals or heat.

THE PROBLEM: *Hair is lighter at the ends.* What you're seeing is the medulla, the inner core of the hair. The only recourse is cutting off the ends.

THE PROBLEM: *Hair snaps.* If your hair breaks midstrand, that's the final straw. Show your stylist the damage, and be prepared to be told you need a serious pruning and a break from chemical processing.

Highlights 101

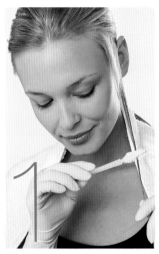

TEST COLOR

Toss the cap and applicator that come with the kit — a clean mascara wand from the beauty-supply store will look more natural. Mix the dye, drape a towel over your shoulders, and determine how long you need for the color to set by brushing it onto a test strand and waiting five minutes. Wipe with a damp cloth, blow-dry, and check. If it's too light, try another strand and check after two minutes. If it's brassy, the color hasn't fully developed; apply more to the area, wait one minute, and test again. Continue the process until you determine how many minutes are optimal.

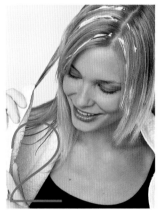

APPLY DYE

Part hair as you normally do, then separate a quarter- to half-inch section above your forehead with a rattail comb, and brush the bleach evenly on both sides from roots to ends (getting as close as possible to the scalp without touching it). Work from the front of your head back: Place one highlight above the middle of your forehead and one on each side above the outer corners of your eyes, followed by two in front of each ear and, finally, three alternating along each side of the part on top.

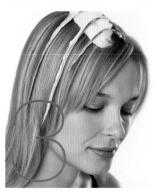

CHECK HAIR

After the allotted time (based on your test in step one), check the color of the first section you painted by wiping it away with a damp towel and blow-drying. If the color looks right, go ahead and rinse your entire head thoroughly with warm water, then wash hair with a shampoo and conditioner designed for color-treated hair. A natural-looking head of highlights is lightest in the front, so don't worry if the strands in the back aren't as bright.

The 10 Commandments

1
Sign language works better than words with stylists. Point to exactly where you want hair to fall.

2
Fine hair looks thicker when it's cut shoulder length or shorter.

3
Naturally wavy hair needs jagged ends to keep it from getting too bushy.

4
To prevent the Bozo look, grow curly hair at least to your shoulders.

5
Long hair shouldn't extend past your breasts.

6
Bangs are universally flattering — unless you have cowlicks or tight curls.

7
For believable blond highlights, ask for up to five different shades of color.

8
If you decide to go brown, do it gradually to keep from ending up too dark.

9
If you hate your new cut or color, talk to the salon manager — most mistakes can be fixed.

10
Sometimes the only cure for damaged, split, or fried hair is a sharp pair of scissors.

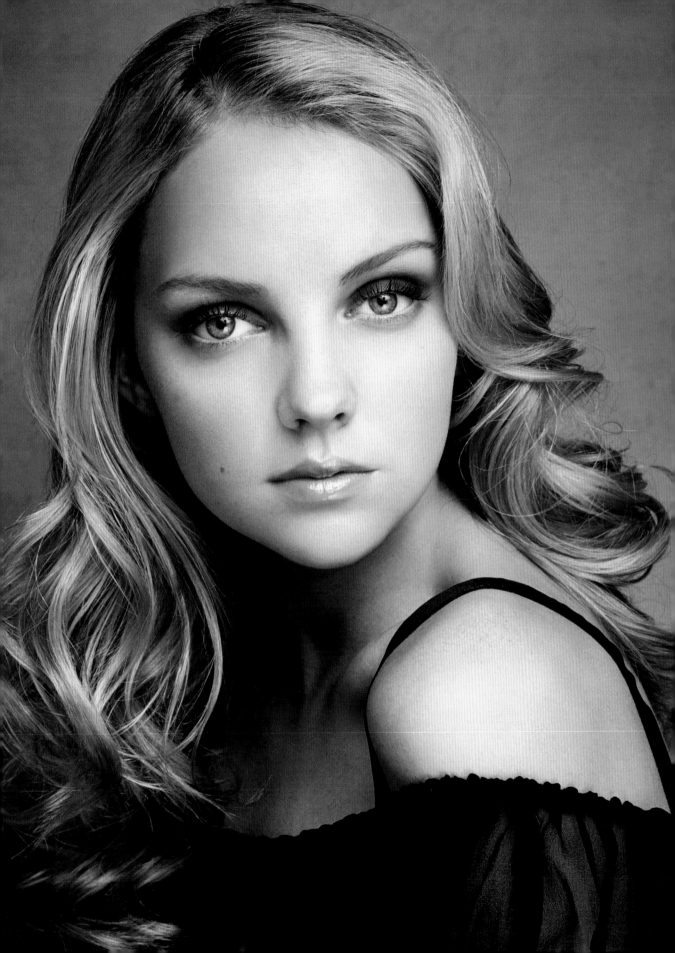

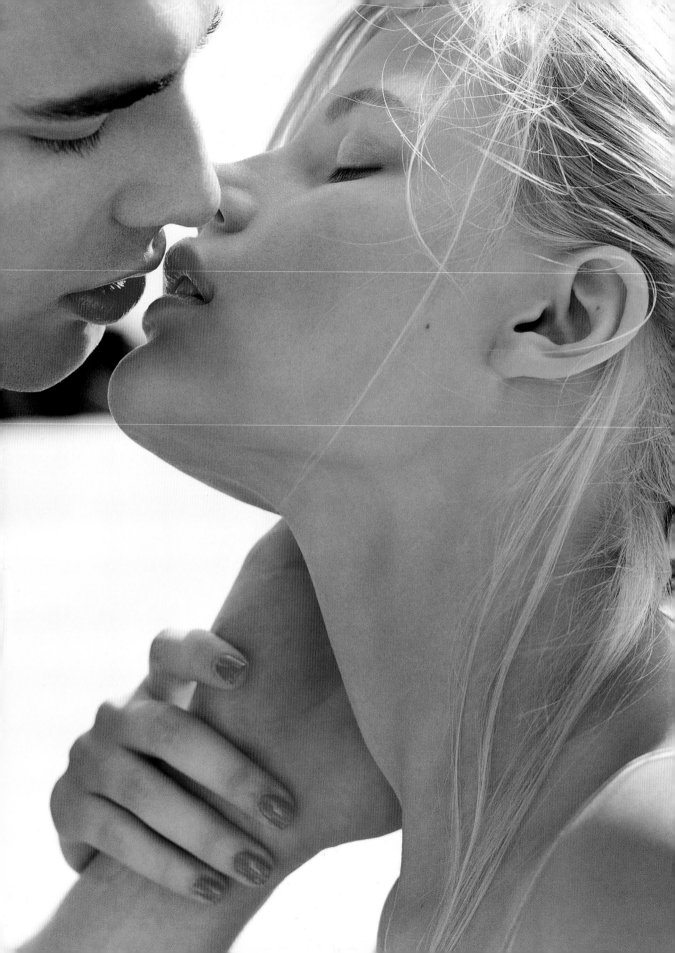

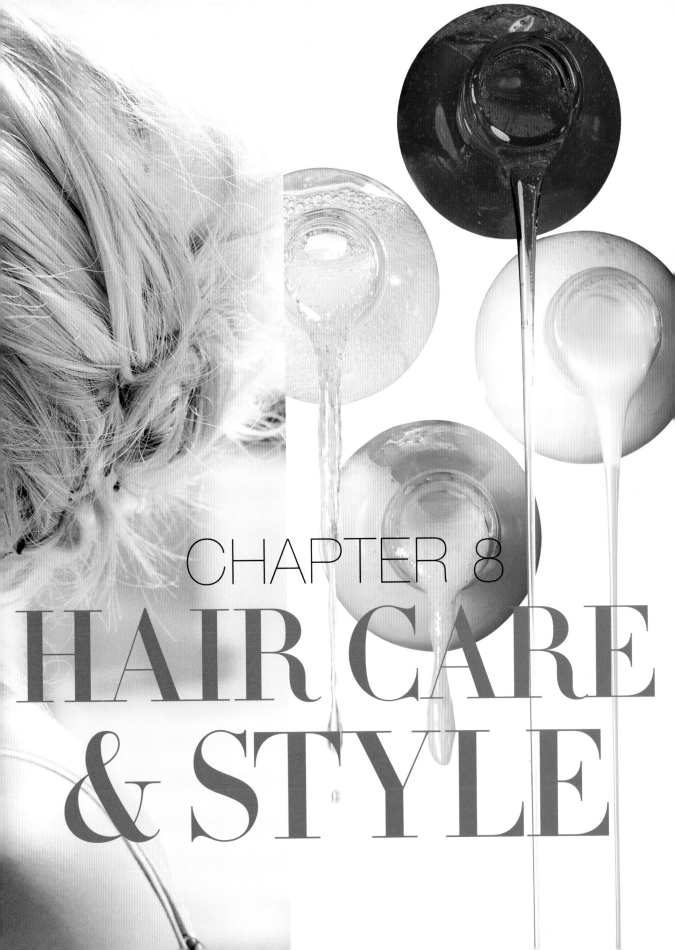

CHAPTER 8
HAIR CARE
& STYLE

Every summer, I throw a party at the beach with saffron-colored cushions in the sand, paper lanterns on poles, a steel-drum band, and lobsters. One year, I decided to get myself decked out, too. I booked hair and makeup pros, and as they fussed over me and gossiped, my husband appeared on the scene. He watched this circus for a few minutes and then asked the obvious question: "Aren't we having a beach party?" Yes, indeed, and this year I was going to be ready.

The minute I stepped on the sand, the wind whipped my hairstyle into a tangled mess, and the humidity evaporated any volume I'd achieved. Even the paper lanterns were nearly shredded. The party was a success, but my labor-intensive look didn't make it past "Day-O." I hate to admit it, but my husband was right. Lobsters and hair mousse don't mix.

As much as I love hair and makeup, there are places where the effort just doesn't pay off, where the elements and the activity conspire against the strongest hair spray. The list includes the beach, ski slopes, and horseback cattle drives. There's no point in fighting it: Gale-force winds are even more powerful than a whole can of Aqua Net.

I thought of this when I met a woman on the beach in Antigua who asked me for a little beauty advice. Her hair was possessed by the humidity, she said, and there was nothing she could do to keep it from frizzing out of control. This I could handle: "Have you tried coating it with conditioner and whirling it into a bun for the day? When you unwind it, your hair will form cascading curls," I said, reciting the tips from a recent story in *Allure.* "Yes. Tried that. Didn't like it," she replied. After rattling off a few other suggestions and getting nowhere, I offered my final piece of wisdom: "Well, you could learn to love your hair." The woman stared at me as if I were from Mars, and said, "Thanks for nothing." Some people seem to prefer being miserable rather than giving in to the elements, even the elements of a tropical paradise.

At the beach, any attempt at artifice or concealment is obvious and jarring. In this perfectly casual domain, flaws can't be hidden. But they can be ignored. What I love about our summer beach party is its release from the formality of so many New York events, where multiple jewels, perfect lipstick, and sky-high stilettos are the norm. Letting your hair blow wild and your feet sink into the sand is what a vacation is about. And for a few carefree hours, what's not to love?

We've learned to accept the truth.

Your mother has told you this, and so has your shrink: Sometimes when you have to fight so hard to make something work, it's better just to let go. Turns out this timeless bit of advice is equally applicable to hair.

DON'T FIGHT YOUR NATURAL TEXTURE. Yes, for special occasions, stick-straight hair can be sizzled into spirals, and ringlets can be blasted into submission with a blow-dryer and a round brush. But for every day, consider working *with* your hair instead of against it, thereby freeing up time that can be spent furthering world peace (or killer abs).

START STYLING IN THE SHOWER. When you know which shampoos and conditioners to use (and how often to use them), hair suddenly snaps to attention and starts behaving. Because many, if not most, women misdiagnose their own hair type, it's important to ask your stylist for an expert opinion. You may think that you have thick hair, but actually have massive amounts of fine strands, or you may believe your hair is dry when it's really your scalp that is.

Limp hair can be brought to life.

"BABY FINE" SOUNDS SO PRETTY — until things go awry, and synonyms like "lank," "flat," and "floppy" seem more apt. Here's how to put the emphasis back on "fine."

WOMEN WITH LIMP HAIR have an excellent excuse for being cheap: Many inexpensive shampoos are actually perfect for your hair because of their higher levels of detergent. When lathered only at the scalp, they wash away excess oil that weighs hair down — and might even allow you to skip a day in between. Wash the length of the hair with a different, more moisturizing formula to keep from completely annihilating your color job, then apply a lightweight rinse-out conditioner only to the ends.

ANOTHER AREA FOR SCRIMPING: styling products. Go easy on gels, sprays, and silicone serums, which can end up plastering your hair to your head. Hairstylists says the real secret to fuller hair is lifting sections up and spraying or smearing mousse or volumizer on the roots before drying.

Beauty 911

At the end of the day, your formerly full-bodied hair is as limp as cold spaghetti.

Go to the bathroom, wet your fingers, and massage the roots of your hair. Then stand in front of an electric hand-dryer, flip your head over, and blow your hair forward while getting some heat on the scalp — allowing hair to cool before flipping it back again. If you are stuck at your desk, pull hair into a butterfly clip on top of the head, mist a bit of aerosol hair spray on the roots, wait for it to dry, then brush hair upside down. The alcohol in the spray will help any oiliness that is making things fall flat.

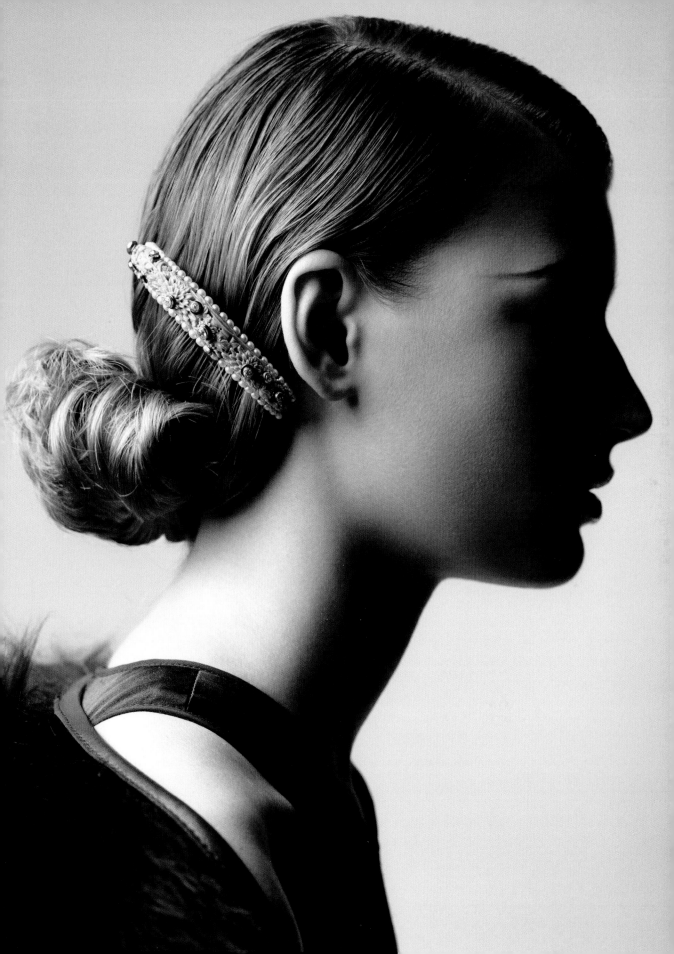

MANY OF US WITH FLAT HAIR have made the mistake of overworking it with the blow-dryer in the pursuit of volume. Set the dryer on low or medium heat, and move it through the roots for just a few minutes, flipping hair upside down or in the opposite direction of how you wear it.

Frizz is our mortal enemy.

Back slowly away from the blow-dryer. It turns out that battling frizz is a matter of keeping your cool, not blasting hair with heat.

GOOD NEWS FOR US SLOPPY TYPES: You really can't overcondition frizzy hair. Shampoo every second or third day with a moisturizing formula, then slick on a rich conditioner (look for words like "deep" or "extra moisture" on the label), and wait at least five minutes before rinsing it out. The heavier conditioning ingredients will coat the cuticle and block out frizz-inducing moisture from the air.

AS SOON AS YOU STEP OUT of the shower, even well-conditioned hair will frizz without a leave-in product to seal the cuticle and lock out moisture. Stylists suggest a one-two punch of smoothing cream and alcohol-free gel. Coarse or curly hair requires two parts cream to one part gel; a ratio of more gel to less cream is better for straight hair. The total blob should be no bigger than a walnut (make that a hazelnut if your hair is chin length or shorter). Rub the mixture between your hands to create a thin film before applying it first from the midpoint to the ends, then distributing from roots to ends with a wide-tooth comb.

ONCE THE BLOW-DRYER IS TURNED ON, there's no turning back — heat will only compound frizz if the hair is left even slightly damp. If you

The Five-Step Plan to Healthy Hair

We once walked into a fellow editor's office and found her in what appeared to be a state of religious ecstasy. Turned out she hadn't found salvation, but rather a split end that had frayed a record-setting eight times. When hair is so damaged that it snaps or splits that dramatically, you need to take steps to save it.

1. Lay off the chemicals.

Even the strongest hair can't withstand a full-on assault of peroxide and straightening solution. Talk to your stylist or colorist about how to give it a rest for at least three months (it may require a different cut or daily routine to camouflage roots or unwanted waves).

2. Shampoo gently.

Hair that's weak or damaged needs a moisturizing shampoo. Wash as infrequently as possible, and unless hair is filthy, there's no need to scrub hard — just rub shampoo into the scalp, and let the runoff clean the ends.

3. Don't stint on conditioner.

Those weekly deep treatments some consider a luxury are now a necessity for you. Consider slathering them on every other day before shampooing (to fill in cracks), then following the wash with a regular rinse-out formula.

4. Protect yourself.

If you can't lay off the blow-dryer completely, at least minimize further damage. Coat strands with a protective styling product, wait until hair is mostly dry (so you spend less time under the nozzle), use the warm setting instead of hot, keep the dryer six inches from the head, and don't point it on one area for too long. If you insist on flatironing, coat hair first with a leave-in conditioner or silicone-based product.

5. Stay out of the sun.

UV rays dry out hair and ruin its color. Before going outside, douse your hair with a leave-in sunscreen treatment — or better yet, wear a hat.

Cheater's Guide

Allure editors are so good at masking unwashed hair, you'd think our pay got docked every time we hit the shampoo bottle. Having finally gotten the message from stylists that most hair looks and feels better if it isn't washed every day, we've come up with all sorts of strategies for stretching the time between shampoos. If hair falls flat overnight, spray it with a volumizer, and push it up and back with a pair of sunglasses before you leave the house; when you get to work, take them down and — presto — extra body. If you wake up to a head of frizz, mist with a protective serum, and clamp a flatiron on small sections at a time, moving quickly to minimize heat damage.

Beauty Myth

The Myth: Wearing hats or tight braids makes hair thinner over time.

THE TRUTH: Unless the hat is so tight that you're cutting off circulation to the hair follicle, there's no reason that growth should be affected. If you repeatedly braid your hair or wear it in a tight ponytail, you risk some breakage — but the hair that grows in will still be healthy.

BEAUTY SCHOOL
Blowout 101

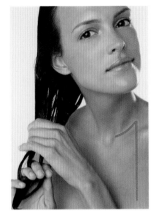

WASH AND LOAD

Shampoo hair, and apply conditioner to the ends only to retain volume. Rinse well, blot excess water with a towel, and massage roots with a nickel-size dab of mousse or volumizer (for fine hair) or a golf-ball-size blob of anti-frizz gel, styling cream, or leave-in conditioner (for dry or puff-prone hair), and comb through. Dry hair for two to three minutes on low speed and high heat; for extra volume, flip hair upside down. Clip the top layers at the crown.

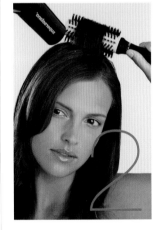

DRY SECTIONS

Gather a two-inch section of hair from the back of the head in a large brush. Hold the dryer — still set on low speed and high heat — about two inches above the roots, and point the nozzle downward. Applying tension, pull the brush and dryer along the length of the hair, lifting it up at the roots and bending it under at the ends. Repeat until the back layers are dry, then reclip so the sides hang down. Repeat the process on the sides, tugging hair up and away from the scalp for volume.

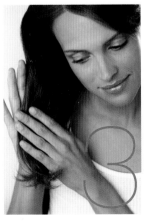

SMOOTH AND FINISH

Gradually unclip the top layers, and don't part hair. Working in two-inch sections, roll the brush as you follow with the dryer, but don't curl ends under (to avoid helmet head). Once hair is dry, part it with comb or fingers. For long, wavy, or coarse hair, rub a dime-size dot of shine serum over the ends only. For fine or normal textures, spritz hair spray on palms, and run them over hair. Tousle with fingers if the style looks too prim and perfect.

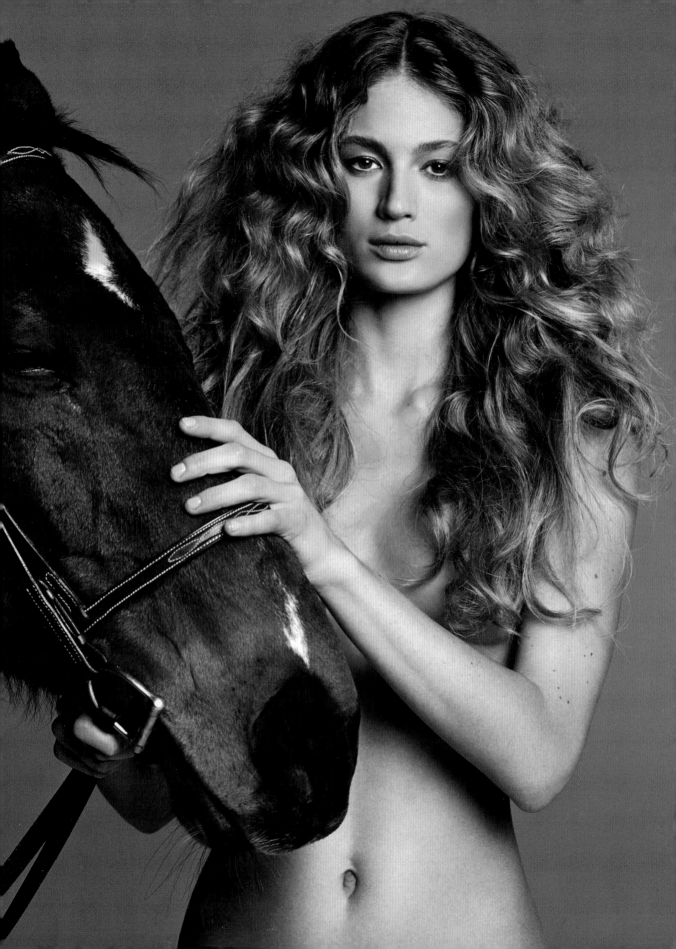

don't have the time or inclination, just apply the styling cocktail, and refrain from touching hair while it air-dries. If you do blow-dry, pull hair taut with a flat brush as you direct the dryer's nozzle from roots to ends. Any last remnants of frizz can be tamed with a few drops of a silicone-based shine serum. Rub it in your palms first, then press onto hair, working from the ends up to avoid overdosing the scalp.

Curl power just needs to be harnessed.

Remember how your mother used to yell at you for constantly flipping and flinging your hair around? If it's curly, she had a point. Unless you want a frazzled mess, waves should largely be left alone.

CONTRARY TO POPULAR BELIEF, curly hair isn't always dry — its cuticle is just more susceptible to being disturbed, which can make strands look dull. Since many shampoos only exacerbate this problem, stick to low-lathering ones that don't contain sulfates (check the label), and wash hair every second or third day. Be sure to follow with a rich, rinse-out conditioner after every shampoo.

THE LESS YOU MESS WITH CURLS, the better they'll look. Since friction causes frizz, don't towel-dry; instead, gently squeeze out excess water with paper towels (they can get closer to the scalp), finger-comb, and rub in a styling cream designed specifically for curl enhancement. Unless you like the Top Ramen look, stay away from any products that contain alcohol — they create crunchy, rigid curls.

CURLS ARE BEST LEFT UNMOLESTED by the dryer. Instead, twist the upper layers around your finger from the root, place each exactly where you want it, and then don't touch the hair until it's dry. If it's the dead of winter and you have to leave in five minutes, at least use a dryer with a diffuser, and move that, not your hands, through your hair.

For dry hair, we try a little tenderness.

Dry hair is like a roof in need of repair: Too much blow-drying, brushing, or chemical processing can cause the cuticle, which should lie flat, to lift up and expose the inner shaft. The result? No, not leaks — dullness, split ends, and a generally fuzzy appearance.

WASH WITH A GENTLE SHAMPOO (specifically labeled for dry or damaged tresses) no more than every other day. Don't pile your hair on your head and wash the whole heap. Just work the shampoo into the scalp and then pat down the rest with excess lather. Conditioning for at least three minutes after every shampoo can also help smooth the cuticle.

Trick of the Trade

If you pick up a 99-cent styling product in an effort to save a few bucks, be warned that cheap formulas are often more concentrated. Stylists suggest applying them sparingly, and only while hair is damp.

WHILE BLOW-DRYING DOESN'T DO DRY HAIR any favors, it's not enemy number one — you just need to prepare hair beforehand. A rich leave-in conditioner (which is a good idea even on air-drying days) mixed with a few drops of silicone serum should do the trick.

EVEN IF YOU TAKE ALL THE PRECAUTIONS in the world, split ends are inevitable. While the only real cure is a trim, you can glue ends back together for a few hours by pinching them with a bit of styling paste (the thick, waxy kind that comes in tins) before smoothing with a tight-bristled brush.

There really isn't a cute euphemism for "greasy."

Those of us with oily hair can only marvel as we hear friends talk about washing their hair every three days. Our hair needs considerably harsher discipline.

WASH OILY HAIR EVERY DAY with a shampoo that contains no extra moisturizing ingredients — a formula for dry or damaged hair is a recipe for lank, greasy disaster. Look for keywords like "balancing" or "anti-residue." Afterward, a light conditioner (or just a little detangler) should be applied only to the ends, never to the roots.

OUT OF THE SHOWER, those who can should avoid applying products at the scalp and steer clear of oil- or silicone-based serums and waxes altogether. Those who need a boost at the roots can achieve it with spray volumizers — the least greasy options. For soft hold all over, choose a lightweight gel.

IF YOU STILL DEVELOP AN OIL SLICK by midday despite these precautions, consider dry shampoo. Sprinkle or spray a little on the roots, and then brush it through the hair to mop up the mess.

Trick of the Trade

Water may be the source of life, but for hair it can be the source of strife. The chlorine in tap water is drying, and the minerals — notably calcium and iron — in hard water build up on hair, making it feel rough and leeching color. To remove chlorine, the pros recommend installing a standard water filter on your showerhead; to reduce mineral content, look for a filter that is also designed to soften water. The difference may amaze you.

Beauty Myth

The Myth: Egg yolks, olive oil, mayonnaise, or avocado make the best deep conditioners.

THE TRUTH: While fatty foods and oils may mimic the feeling of moisture, they just sit on hair, making it greasy and flat. The lightweight emulsions in store-bought conditioners will smooth the cuticle more evenly — and they don't leave behind a sticky (or stinky) residue.

We're not saying we have dandruff, but if we did, you'd never know.

This may be small consolation, but those unsightly flakes aren't a consequence of bad behavior. Dandruff is an inflammatory skin condition caused by a common yeast called *Pityrosporum ovale,* and it *can* be controlled, if not cured.

AT THE FIRST SIGN OF SNOW, start using a drugstore dandruff shampoo every time you wash your hair (at least three to five times a week). Ingredients to look for are sulfur, zinc pyrithione, selenium sulfide, salicylic acid, or tar — and fortunately, more and more shampoo makers are now packing them in less repugnant, conditioning formulas. Flakes can usually be brought under control within two to four weeks, at which point you can wash with that shampoo just once a week. Because dandruff shampoos tend to be drying, be sure to slather on an extra-rich rinse-out conditioner afterward.

STYLING PRODUCTS DON'T EXACERBATE the yeast that causes dandruff. That said, retire any gels, mousses, and hair sprays that make the problem look worse. If there's any alcohol in them, they're more likely to flake.

Deep-conditioning treatments aren't just a slick marketing gimmick.

Having grown up watching those commercials for hot-oil treatments, we thought the whole idea seemed a little old fashioned — until we talked to a few cosmetics chemists. They told us deep conditioners really do penetrate the hair and strengthen from the inside out. Not bad for a few minutes' work.

START BY CHOOSING THE RIGHT FORMULA for your hair — the coarser your strands, the richer and creamier the consistency should be. Start with dry, unwashed hair, and massage your scalp with your fingertips to loosen dead skin and spread natural sebum uniformly. Then wet hair, and squeeze out excess water with a towel until it's damp.

MASSAGE QUARTER-SIZE BLOBS of conditioner into one-inch sections of hair, starting a half inch down from the roots, and distribute through with a wide-tooth comb. Then cover hair with a shower cap, and blast a hair-dryer over the cap to open the cuticle and increase absorption. Wait (as patiently as you can) for three to ten minutes, depending on how damaged your hair is.

RINSE OUT MOST OF THE CONDITIONER, until hair feels clean and not too slick, then shampoo once (or even twice, if you've really globbed it on) to remove any residue. Finish with a dose of your regular daily conditioner. The experts recommend you go through this little routine once a month, or every two weeks if your hair is really fried. We tried it, and now we're believers.

Beauty Myth

The Myth: Lather, rinse, repeat.

THE TRUTH: We blame this one on TV commercials from our youth. The truth is that shampooing hair more than once a day — never mind twice in a single shower — strips hair of the natural oils necessary for shine and overall lusciousness. You only need to shampoo once and rinse until water runs clear and hair no longer feels sudsy.

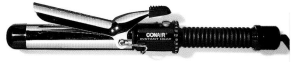

There's a right way and a wrong way to use a curling iron.

We still have affectionate memories of that little butane-powered curling iron we brought to school for touch-ups. But today's irons are bigger and better — and we now know not to roll up our entire head into sausage curls.

FOR THE MOST NATURAL-LOOKING, RELAXED CURL, choose an iron with a barrel that is at least one and a half inches in diameter. (Only women with exceptionally fine hair should use a one-inch barrel.)

AFTER DRYING HAIR SMOOTH with a round brush, use the iron just from ear level down. Then, instead of clipping the curling iron onto the ends and rolling hair up, apply this technique favored by top stylists: Hold the iron vertically instead of horizontally, wrap a one-inch section around the barrel, and pull the piece taut with your fingers (instead of the clamp) for about five seconds. Your results will be more realistic than perfect Cindy Brady ringlets if you don't curl the ends.

IF YOU HAVE THICK HAIR, pin up the top layer, and curl the underside first, being careful not to disturb each coil once it's released, then unpin and finish the top. Once the waves have cooled, muss them up a bit with your fingers (not a brush, which can wreck new curls).

Guilty as Charged

We'd rather not live without our flatiron.

We have a love-hate relationship with our flatirons. No styling implement is more damaging to hair — or more addictive. Since some use them practically every day even though we know better, we figured we'd better ask the top stylists how to minimize the carnage. They all recommended that you choose a model with a ceramic, not metal, plate, which glides over hair better, causes less friction, and distributes the heat more evenly. Then be sure that hair is 100 percent, totally dry first and that strands are liberally coated with a heat-protective spray before you clamp them down. Finally, read that boring little instruction booklet that comes in the box: Clinical studies have shown that you can minimize damage by leaving the iron on each section of hair for no longer than the manufacturer's recommended time.

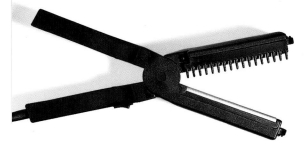

Trick of the Trade

A small tube of hand lotion in your purse can bail you out of hair trouble. In the summer, running a tiny amount through your hair with your fingertips can tame frizz. Come winter, rub a smidgen on your hands, then smooth them over the head to eliminate static.

Brushing Up

ROUND
GOOD FOR: Creating tension to straighten hair; building volume at the root

DOWNSIDE: If used when blow-drying ends, can create an undesirable flip or curl; can easily get tangled in hair

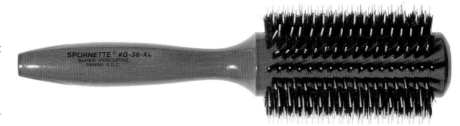

OVAL
GOOD FOR: Drying the length of the hair and finishing the ends

DOWNSIDE: Can't create as much volume at the root as a round brush

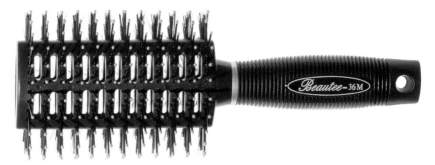

VENTED
GOOD FOR: Combing through wet or semidry hair

DOWNSIDE: Vents prevent the brush from heating up, so straightening is more difficult; air coming through vents can create static

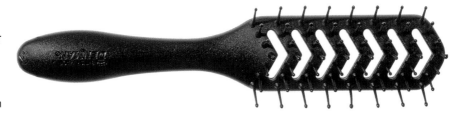

METAL ROUND
GOOD FOR: Setting hair like a roller

DOWNSIDE: If the metal heats up too much, it can damage fragile hair

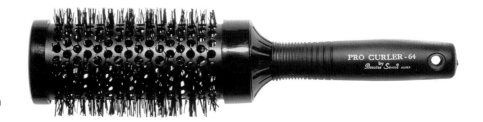

PADDLE
GOOD FOR: Finishing ends

DOWNSIDE: Can't create volume

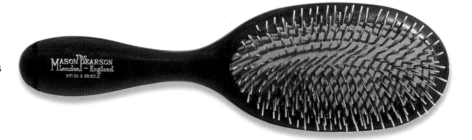

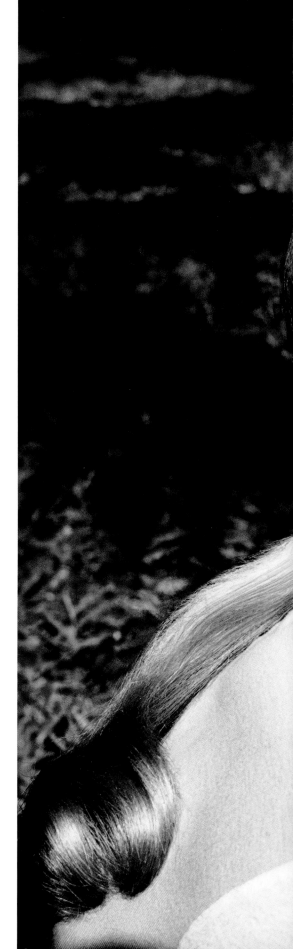

We've learned how to make even a plain ponytail look elegant.

When it comes to the world's easiest hairstyle, placement is everything: Anchor the ponytail either all the way up on the crown or down at the nape of the neck. You may think you're playing it safe by sticking to the middle, but the result is less stylish and more "I'm off to the gym."

HIGH PONYTAILS BENEFIT FROM A LITTLE TEASING at the crown. Create some height on top by flipping the head over while blow-drying (to add volume overall), then teasing the area that will sit just above the finished ponytail. Sweep hair straight back with no part (but don't pull it too tight), and secure the tail with a snag-free elastic. We then like to tug one lock of hair out from the underside of the ponytail, wrap it around the elastic to cover it, and secure that end with a bobby pin. The result is sophisticated enough for pretty much any event.

FOR LOW PONYTAILS, the key is a deep part and lots of shine. Spread a small blob of styling gel between your hands, run them through dry hair until it's shiny, then part hair on one side — the deeper the part, the more dramatic the look — and secure it with a snag-free elastic. If hair is shoulder length or shorter, just pull it through the elastic one and a half times, leaving the ends sticking up and the tail looped against the nape of your neck. Finish by pinching the ends with a waxy pomade to keep them neat.

Trick of the Trade

To smooth flyaways at the hairline, try a little trick favored by runway stylists: Mist a toothbrush with hair spray, and sweep back the tiny hairs. The effect lasts for several hours.

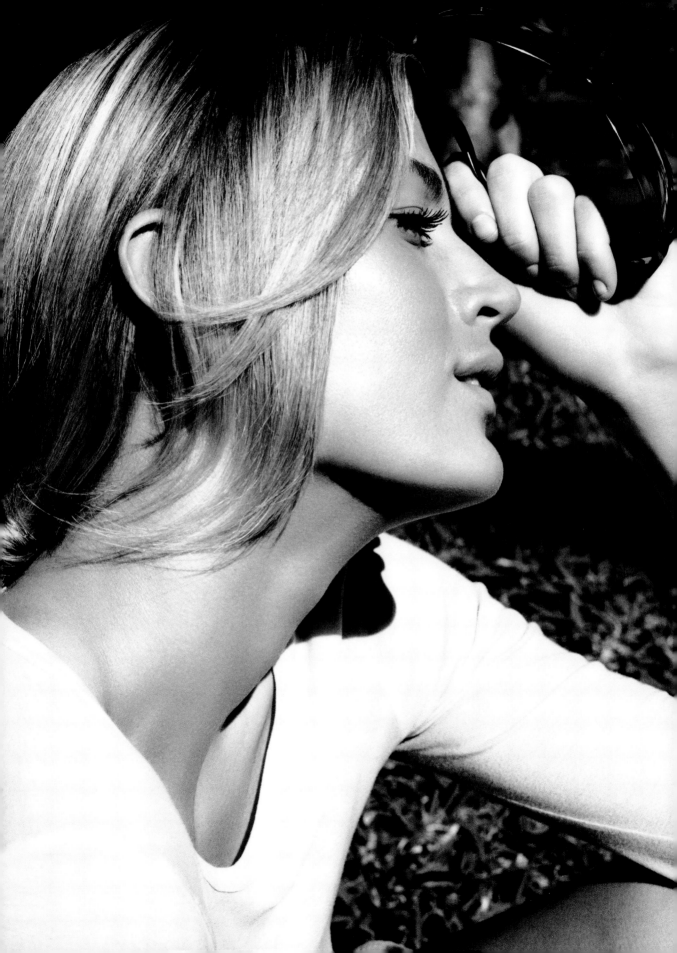

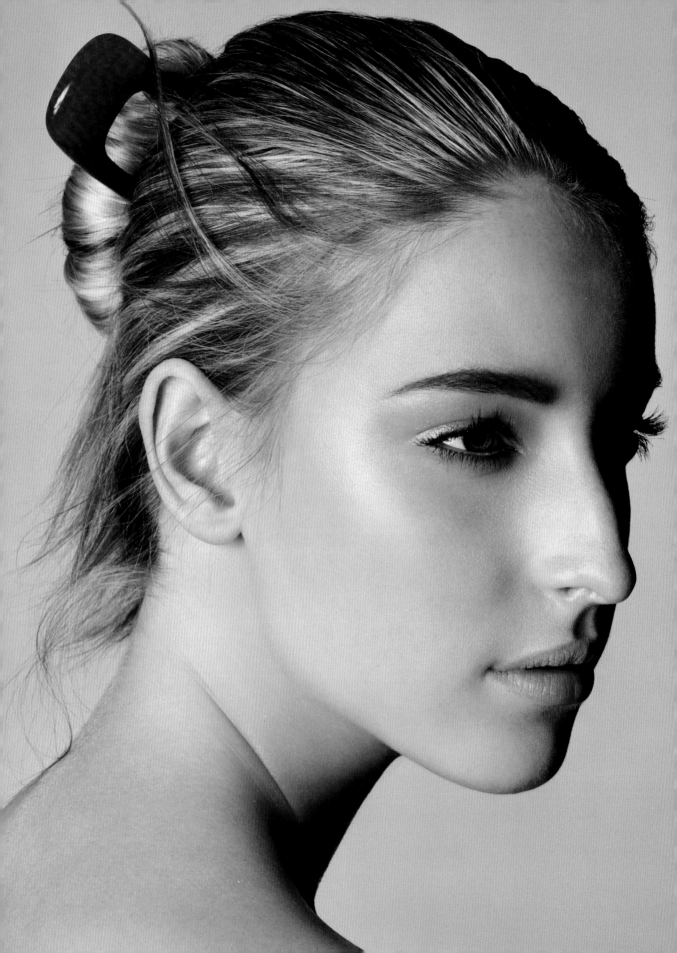

Updos aren't just for the prom anymore.

Forget champagne: The surest sign of a truly big night out is when we make the effort to wear our hair up. And it can actually be pretty easy to accomplish.

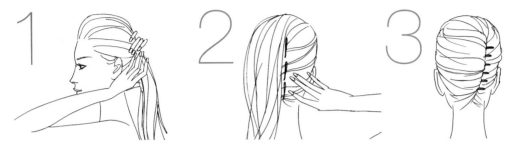

THE FRENCH TWIST HAS GOTTEN A BAD RAP for looking more like a helmet than a hairstyle. But when it's loose and a bit disheveled, the effect is soft and sexy — more Ivanka than Ivana. Start by pulling hair into a ponytail in the middle of the head and twisting it while moving it upward. Then hold the twist against the head so the ends of the hair are pointing up, and insert a few pins into the underside to create an anchor. Fold the ends back down, and tuck them under the twist, pinning along the seam until the twist feels secure (it could take up to ten pins, depending on your length). Then comes the crucial step: Grab a few small sections that are short and on the verge of falling out, and pull them loose. To make sure this undone style stays, mist the tugged pieces lightly with hair spray.

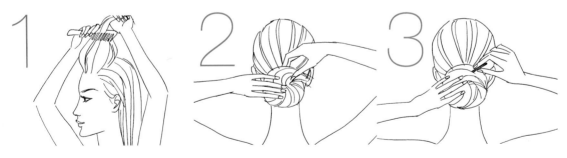

A MODERN TAKE ON THE CLASSIC BUN is easy — as long as you have enough hair to gather into a ponytail that's at least three inches long. Draw a part two inches off center with a comb. At the back of the part, drag the comb down toward one ear, then the other, so hair is divided into three sections. Then take the left and right sides, bring them together at the back of the head — level with the earlobes — and secure in a loose ponytail with an elastic. Finish by grabbing the miniponytail and bringing it up and over the elastic. Tuck the ends into the elastic so it forms a small, tight loop, then push four or five bobby pins into the sides of the loop so they're hidden.

The 10 Commandments

1

Lather, rinse, and don't bother repeating. It's unnecessary.

2

Only those with truly oily hair should wash it every day.

3

Don't fight your natural texture — work with it.

4

To give limp hair a boost, steer clear of everything but light volumizers.

5

The less you mess with curls, the better.

6

To fight frizz, load up on conditioner and a mix of styling cream and gel.

7

If you have dry hair, deep-condition it regularly.

8

The best ponytails are anchored either up high on the head or down low on the neck.

9

Big-barrel curling irons yield the most natural-looking waves.

10

If you must use a flatiron, minimize damage by using it on dry, never damp, hair.

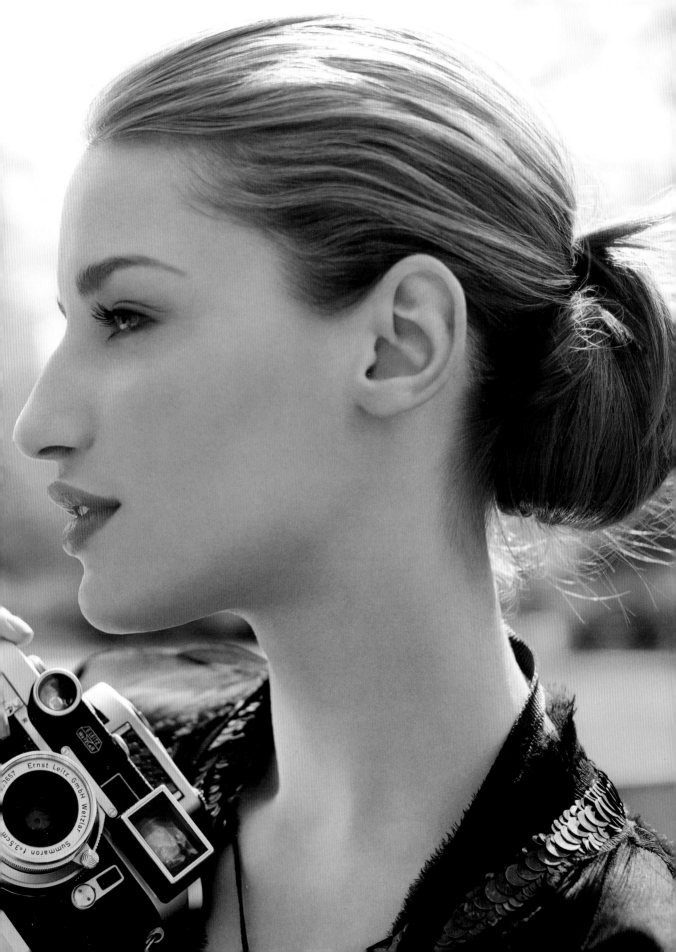

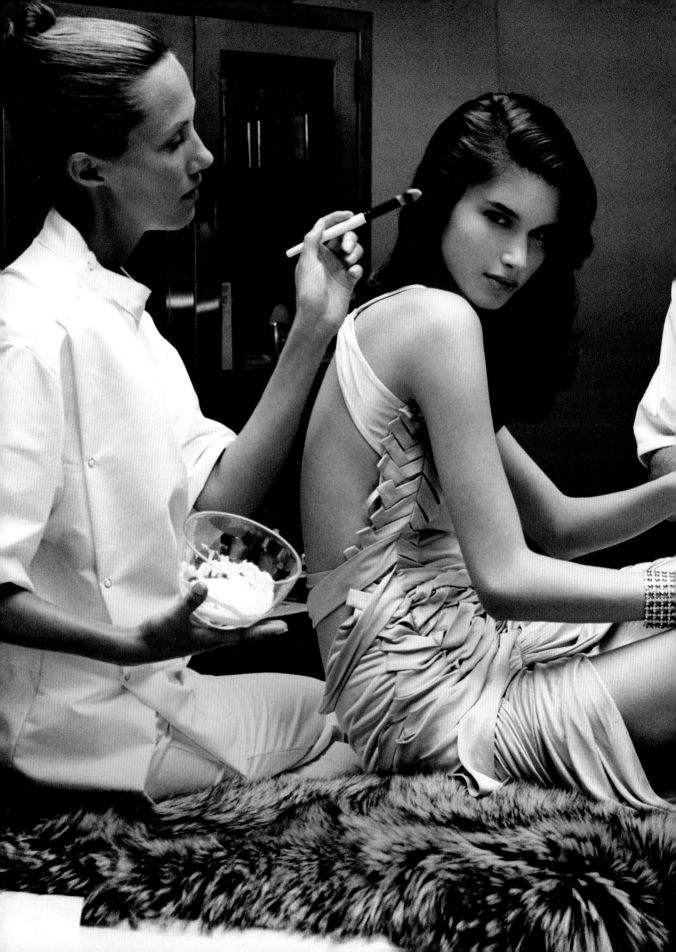

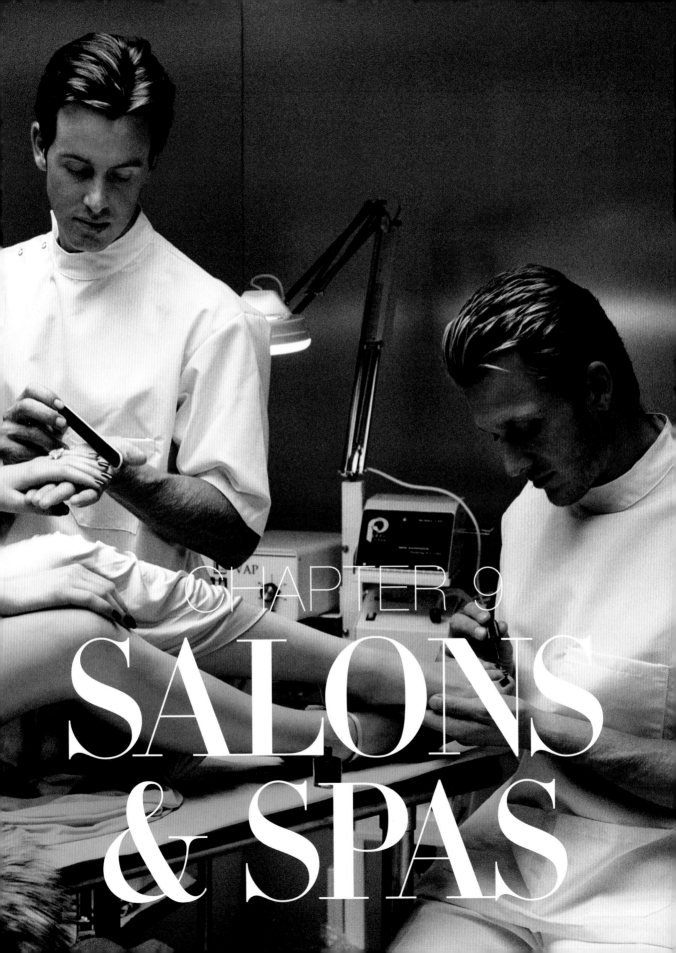

CHAPTER 9

SALONS & SPAS

I was introduced to beauty salons by my mother, who used to take me with her when she got her hair done (my mother's hair was always "done," not cut, not styled, and never colored). I would read magazines while René would roll my mother's hair in big curlers and then release fat ringlets that he'd comb and tease into an airy soufflé. The place was always buzzing. Women would sit under helmet hair-dryers with cotton in their ears, smoking cigarettes and chatting over the din. It was a foreign land with its own rituals, costume, and language, and it was a mystery to me.

When I got a little older, my mother talked me into submitting my own long, lank hair to René or Monsieur Marc or one of those other doting men with no last name. I'd put a robe over my shirt, stick my neck in the guillotine-like sink, and then beg for just a trim, not a cut, never a hairdo. At that very moment, René or Marc would suddenly lose the ability to understand English. They'd indulge me with the sweetest smile and then whack off four inches, telling me I looked marvelous.

I have since learned to navigate the salon as well as my mother does. I now know to remove my shirt before putting on the robe so that the collar doesn't get in the way of the cut, how to chat with the receptionist, shampooer, and manicurist, and to slip each one a tip without breaking eye contact. Most of all, I've found my own one-named stylist, whom I trust as if he were performing bypass surgery every six weeks. When he suggests a change, I rarely object; I can't even remember the last time I said the words "Just a trim."

Over the years, I've also figured out how to request a silent massage, how to read a magazine while getting a manicure, and how to resist a facialist's product pitch while she examines my skin disapprovingly. Some things are still a mystery, though. No matter how many times someone heralds a particular bikini waxer's work as painless, I continue to find the process excruciating. I haven't figured out how to stand stark naked for an airbrush tanning session without unspeakable embarrassment. And I still can't summon the patience for a relaxation treatment that lasts longer than a movie. A day of beauty, to me, is about ten hours too long.

We know how to score the best appointments (without dropping any names).

Yes, it would be mighty easy to get into spas if we just admitted where we work, but we don't. (As anonymous visitors, we can see what the place is *really* like.) As a result, we've spent probably two and a half days of our lives on hold with receptionists, and besides checking our email and doodling, we've used that time to figure out ways to score the best time slots.

BUTTER UP THE RECEPTIONIST. That starts with learning her name and using it every time you call — a shockingly small gesture that nevertheless blows them away at the front desk, since they're typically ignored or berated. Send a thank-you note or even a tiny gift after she gets you on the schedule, and you're pretty much set for life.

BE FLEXIBLE. Midmorning and midafternoon appointments are always going to be more plentiful than lunchtime or Saturday. If you want to see a real A-list stylist, you have to put yourself at the mercy of his schedule. Which means you have to wait.

TRULY DESPERATE TO GET IN THAT DAY? Call the spa or salon five minutes after it opens. That will give them enough time to go through messages from the previous night, and give you first crack at cancellations. If nothing's available, give them your cell number just in case — and turn your ringer on loud. If the scheduler can't reach you, it's on to the next person on the list.

TRY NOT TO CANCEL YOUR OWN APPOINTMENT too often. If you don't give the salon 24 hours' notice, they won't be happy (and may charge

Trick of the Trade

Consider booking appointments in blocks. You can maximize your downtime by, say, getting a manicure while your facial is in progress (and your nails will be totally dry and smudge-proof when it's over). Just be careful not to choose lethal combinations: a postwaxing salt scrub stings like a whole nest of hornets, and snips from a haircut can fall into wet nail polish.

Beauty 911

A lunchtime facial leaves your skin red, blotchy, and greasy — and you have to go back to work.

Don't worry — your boss doesn't have to find out that you weren't really at the doctor. Rinse your face with cool water, and reduce the redness and swelling with a thin layer of 1 percent hydrocortisone cream (not ointment, which will only leave you as slick as a seal). Then even out the blotchiness with a fine layer of powder foundation, which is less likely to clog pores than a cream formula.

you). If you cancel more than twice a year, the salon receptionist may make your life difficult. Same goes for running late. If it's more than ten minutes, call and apologize (and throw in a little groveling for good measure).

We mind our manners.

Your computer file at the salon may be as close as you'll get to an FBI dossier. Salon spies may keep notes on your hair-color formulation — as well as your tipping habits.

BE NICE TO EVERYONE. Besides being good karma, salon staffers talk — and gripe — about customers, and if you're snippy with the girl who washes your hair, it will definitely get back to your stylist.

TURN OFF YOUR PHONE. Not only does yakking irritate stylists, but you aren't likely to pay much attention to the service you're getting — opening you up to nasty surprises when you press End.

SIT SILENTLY, IF YOU PLEASE. You're not required to chat with a stylist or manicurist. We simply tell the pro, "You don't mind if I just zone out, do you? Today has been crazy." Then we close our eyes — the universal sign for "Please don't bore me with the latest rumor about celebrity infidelity."

We've learned that there's no preparing for a spa visit.

No matter how bad our bikini stubble, gnarly our feet, or overgrown our roots, we know the beauty pros have seen far worse. And sometimes you have to let yourself go to get the best results.

FOR THE MOST THOROUGH WAXING, wait until hair is a full quarter inch long. And if you are

Salon Waxing 101

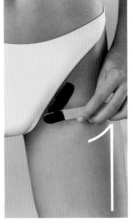

PREPARE YOURSELF

Make sure you have at least a quarter inch of hair growth before your session — the wax needs something to hold on to. And don't pick a day during the week before your period (studies show that's when women are most susceptible to pain). Popping a few ibuprofen an hour before your appointment helps — or if you're really wimpy (like us), apply a numbing cream, but only to small areas like the bikini line.

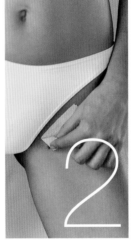

WAX ON, WAX OFF

If you have sensitive skin, make sure the aesthetician uses a wax that contains chamomile — it's the most soothing — and applies it to small sections at a time. (If someone promises they can do a Brazilian in 15 minutes, you know you're in trouble.) Once things are under way, resist the temptation to watch the action; it's much better to breathe steadily and zone out. After each strip, the waxer should press her hand on the skin to stop the pain. If she doesn't, ask her to, or do it yourself.

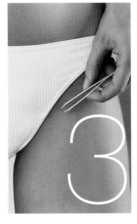

PREVENT INGROWNS

Start exfoliating 24 hours after your appointment. You can use a loofah or a chemical exfoliant — the best ones contain both salicylic acid to unplug pores and glycolic acid to slough off dead skin. To make the next wax easier, consider slathering the area with a hair-minimizing lotion between appointments, and keep your hands off that razor. If you shave, it's back to square one.

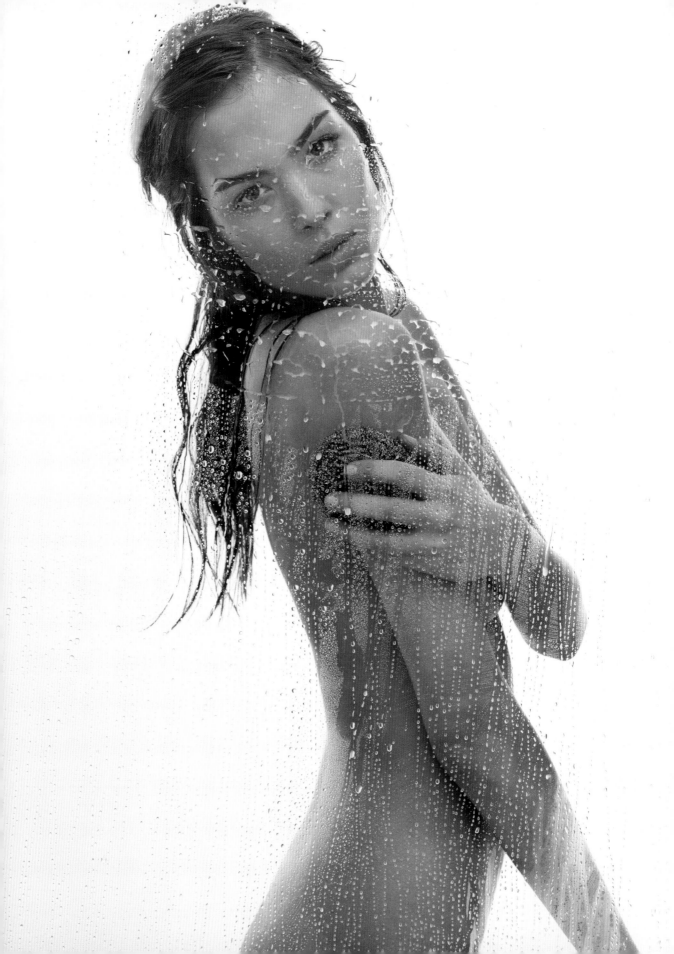

going the laser-hair-removal route, resist the temptation to wax between sessions. Yanking hair out will disturb the follicle, throw off the regrowth cycle, and completely undermine the laser schedule you'd planned so painstakingly.

STEP AWAY FROM THE RAZOR on the day of a body scrub (it will hurt like hell if you don't) and the day after a self-tanning treatment (you'll scrape that fake bronze right off). It's an excellent idea to shave before self-tanning, though — the blade exfoliates dead skin that can cause color to develop unevenly.

FOR A MANICURE AND PEDICURE, don't cut your nails ahead of time. If they're too short, the manicurist can't shape them. Just show up with clean soles and a good book.

We dress the part.

Never mind what you look like lounging around the waiting area. When dressing for a beauty appointment, there are more important concerns than aesthetics.

AT THE HAIR SALON, we take off our shirt before slipping on the robe. Otherwise, a high neckline can get coated with scratchy hairs or stained with dye, and anything bumpy (like a collar) can prevent the stylist from cutting a clean line.

FLIP-FLOPS AREN'T JUST FOR SUMMER — or the beach. The only way to guarantee you don't

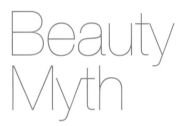

Beauty Myth

The Myth: You need extractions to clean out your pores.

THE TRUTH: A facial can temporarily diminish blackheads, but excessive extractions can actually lead to enlarged pores, especially around the nostrils. It's best to diligently apply creams containing salicylic acid to unplug pores and keep them clean.

Shopping for Steals

Practice makes perfect — and fledgling stylists, colorists, and masseurs need someone to practice on. That's what training nights are for. Salons offer cuts and color from junior stylists at significantly reduced rates, and massage therapy schools arrange for students to knead away for less than the price of a citrus-mint-verbena lotion. To find out how to get on the list, ask your favorite salon (some hold open calls; others have sign-ups). Just be warned that you do have to give up some of the usual luxuries. This includes creative control (many salons require that you be willing to cut at least two inches), time (students watch demonstrations and receive instruction), and privacy (even in a massage, the teachers may come in to watch the session).

smudge your pretty fuchsia pedicure, even after a half hour under those little fans, is to slip on a pair of thongs. If it's 20 degrees outside or raining, wait 30 minutes, then ask the pedicurist to coat your nails with oil and plastic wrap to prevent smudging.

WEAR SWEATS TO YOUR WAXING APPOINTMENT. (If you're coming straight from work, slip them into your bag for later.) Tight pants will chafe newly raw skin and make it more likely to erupt in tiny red bumps.

We speak up if we hate our new look.

Our first instinct is to sit silently, nodding at the stylist, until we can escape and burst into tears on the sidewalk. But that tactic isn't going to help prevent the mess or repair the damage. Here's what will.

IF YOU HATE YOUR NEW CUT, STAY CALM. In fact, when the stylist asks you what you think, avoid words like "hate," "hideous," or "mutilated," and say, "This isn't what I had in mind." Explain the problem, then ask, "Would you please try to fix it?" He should do exactly that, on the spot. If you just don't like the way it was styled, ask for another blow-dry. If you don't have time for a redo, tell the manager on the way out that you aren't happy, but you're going to give it 48 hours to see how things shape up — and that you'll be calling her if they don't. They may offer you a new cut or tweak free of charge, but unless you have a bald spot, you probably won't get the original one comped.

THE SAME GOES FOR COLOR. It may be too harsh to apply more chemicals that day, and it can

Guilty as Charged

We buy products we don't need — or even want.

We like to think we're incredibly tough and savvy . . . and then we get suckered into buying some outrageously priced ointment that the facialist swears on a Bulgarian Bible will totally eliminate broken capillaries. The best way to get out of high-pressure sales situations is simply to say that you have all the products you need right now, so no, thank you. Then there's the actual way we weasel out: Say, "My skin can be really sensitive to new products. I'm going to see how it reacts to what you used today. I'll call you." And then we really make a break for it.

Beauty Myth

The Myth: You have to get naked for a massage.

THE TRUTH: Guess what? You're paying, so you get to decide what stays on or comes off. While a bra actually *will* get in the way, panties are easily shifted down if a masseuse needs to reach your lower back.

be helpful to walk around for a day to see how your hair looks in natural light. But if you aren't pleased, ask the salon to offer an adjustment gratis.

SPA SERVICES ARE ANOTHER STORY. Just because you didn't enjoy your massage doesn't mean you're entitled to a second one to fix the first. However, if the aesthetician was running so late that your body treatment had to be cut short, or if constant racket in the hallway prevented you from being able to relax, speak up. It's best to talk directly to the manager, who's less likely to get defensive — and more likely to offer you a free service to make up for your bad one.

We've learned how to break up with a stylist without tears (his or ours).

Ending a long-term relationship with a hairstylist can be just as messy as any other breakup — and potentially more frightening, considering how sharp those scissors are. But with a little tact, you really can untangle yourself without getting hurt.

Trick of the Trade

Some people believe that bringing a photo to your hairstylist is somehow tacky or insulting. Not so. Celebrity stylist Garren has told us, "Photos give me a direction. They show a client's wish or dream, and then I can tell them if it will work or not." That said, it's nicer to present the picture by saying, "Do you mind if I show you something?" rather than "I want *this*."

CRASH COURSE

Maximizing Your Massage

When you're paying for an hour of knot-busting bliss, you shouldn't have to worry about how to ask for exactly what you want. The masseuse might even be grateful for some direction, rather than having to guess what "unnnnh" and "ooooh" mean.

1 SHOW UP AT LEAST TEN MINUTES BEFORE YOUR APPOINTMENT, which will allow you time to fill out a few forms (if it's your first visit), change, and decompress.

2 GIVE A BRIEF DEBRIEFING. Tell the therapist about any injuries or sensitive spots, and what you'd like her to concentrate on during the session. Ask if she has a shower cap to protect your hair from oils if you aren't going straight home after your appointment. If you'd like silence during the treatment, speak now, saying, "I'm going to just drift off once we start, so is there anything else I need to know?" That doesn't sound like "Shut up" — but it politely conveys the same message. (If she persists, say, "Sorry, I can't talk right now. I'm sooooo relaxed." Who could take offense at a compliment like that?)

3 IF THE PRESSURE IS TOO HARD — OR TOO SOFT — SPEAK UP RIGHT AWAY. Don't assume the therapist can interpret your nonverbal cues. And if you feel too exposed, just say, "Would you please drape me a little more?" It's reasonable to expect every part of your body except the one being worked on to be covered by the sheet.

4 AT THE END OF THE MASSAGE, ASK FOR A TOWEL IF YOU FEEL GREASY. When you get home, drink plenty of water. Massage can release lactic acid that builds up in muscles, causing soreness the next day; water will help flush it from your system.

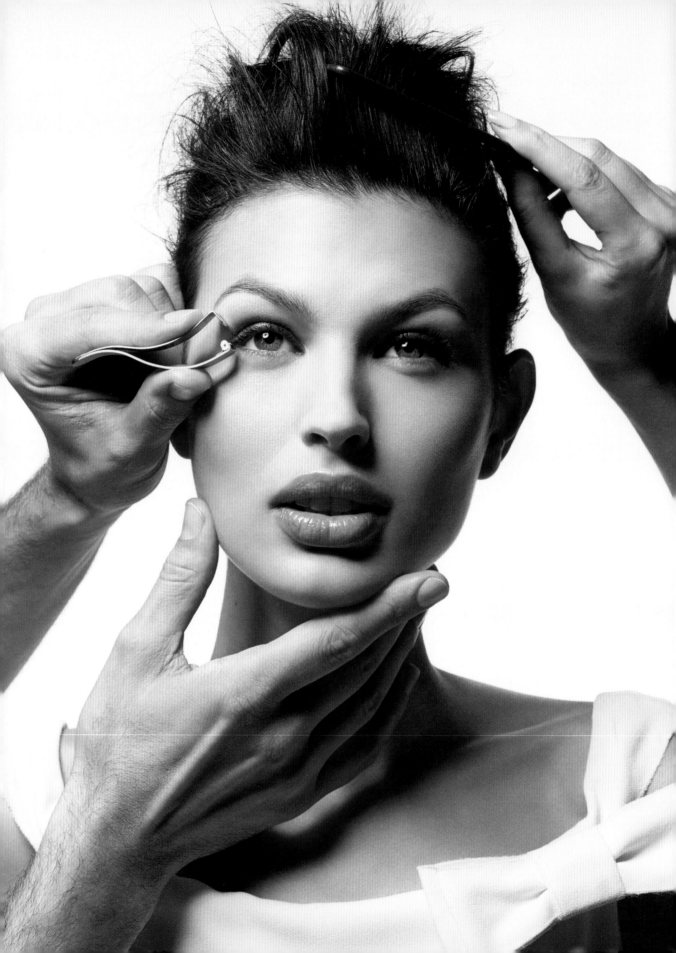

FIRST OFF, DON'T LIE. The old "I'm moving to France" line only guarantees that you will end up behind him at the movies. Instead, start by taking a break. (If you can handle it, tell him your plans. If you can't, move to the next step.)

TRY SOMEONE NEW, and if it's a perfect match, write a sweet, concise note to your old stylist that doesn't go into specifics — something along the lines of "I wanted to let you know that I felt like a change. I wish you well."

IF YOU DECIDE YOU WANT TO RETURN TO YOUR EX, don't pretend you haven't cheated — a good stylist will see through that with one glance at your new layers. Use the moment to voice whatever you're unhappy with, whether it's his three-week waitlist or the fact that you're tired of your chin-length bob. And consider the fact that you might be partially to blame. If you always say, "Just a little trim today," you might be stifling his creativity — and your own.

We've finally figured out the whole tipping thing.

With all those shampooers, coat checkers, and coffee fetchers, spas and salons give most of us a serious case of tipping anxiety. Take a deep breath, and follow these simple guidelines.

THE OVERALL TIP FOR SERVICES should be about 15 percent; you can then scale up or down if you are thrilled or disappointed. These days, many spas encourage you to add the tip to the final bill, and the manager will divvy it up later.

IF YOU WANT A LITTLE MORE CONTROL over who gets what, bring small bills. One salon owner we know recommends $5 for the person who shampooed your hair, $1 for the one who

brought you a cappuccino (maybe $2 if you had a special request, like soy milk), and between $1 and $3 for the coat check.

IF THE PERSON WHO PAINTS YOUR NAILS or cuts your hair owns the joint, you really and truly don't have to tip. (That said, we don't know many owners who actually *refuse* gratuities.) If you feel weird just walking out, consider giving him a present around the holidays — a nice bottle of wine, an orchid, or even a donation to charity in his name all go over well.

A TIP IS A TIP IS A TIP, no matter how you hand it over. Most salons have little manila envelopes at the front desk (just be sure to write a note on the outside and sign your name). But no stylist or aesthetician really minds being handed a neatly folded bill.

Cheater's Guide

As much as we like to plan ahead, we also value spontaneity. An untended bikini line would be a lame reason to decline a last-minute invitation to a friend's beach house. When you need hair gone, stat, depilatory cream is the answer. Not only does it work fast, but it also doesn't cause nicks or stubble. If you have to shave, know that you're about to undo that fine regrowth you've gained through waxing. But hey, it's a beach weekend! What the hell! And while you're feeling all crazy and rebellious, why not try this trick we learned from a very famous porn star: Smooth on an antibiotic ointment like Neosporin instead of soap or cream; it allows the razor to glide easily and takes care of the bacteria that can cause bumps. Shave in the direction of hair growth, and stick with a conservative shape. (We didn't learn that last bit from the porn star.)

The 10 Commandments

1
Get to know the receptionist — she can help you snag an appointment.

2
Those willing to take midday appointments during the week get in faster.

3
Mind your manners, especially with assistants.

4
Massage therapists, stylists, and colorists aren't psychic — tell or show them what you want (and what you don't).

5
To escape mindless chatter, close your eyes. It's the universal sign for silence.

6
Shaving before a wax or clipping your nails before a manicure won't get you the best results.

7
Take ibuprofen an hour before waxing to minimize the pain.

8
If you hate your new cut or color, speak up — you're entitled to a fix.

9
Tip 15 to 20 percent of the bill, and give a few dollars to the coat checker, shampooer, and anyone else who helped you during your visit.

10
If a beauty pro is pushing products you don't want, say you have to think about it.

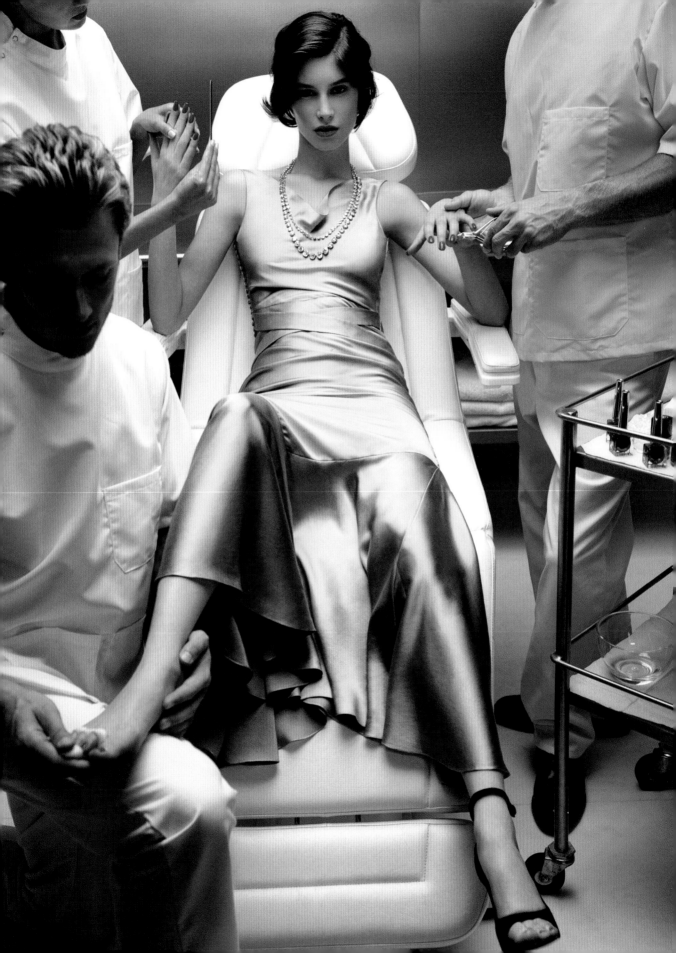

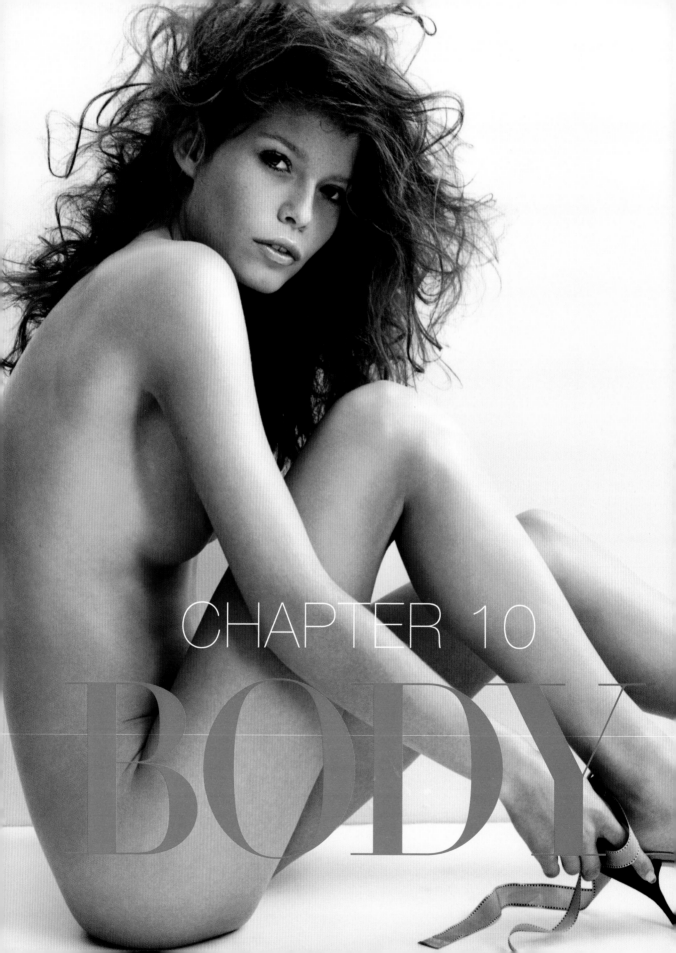

CHAPTER 10

BODY

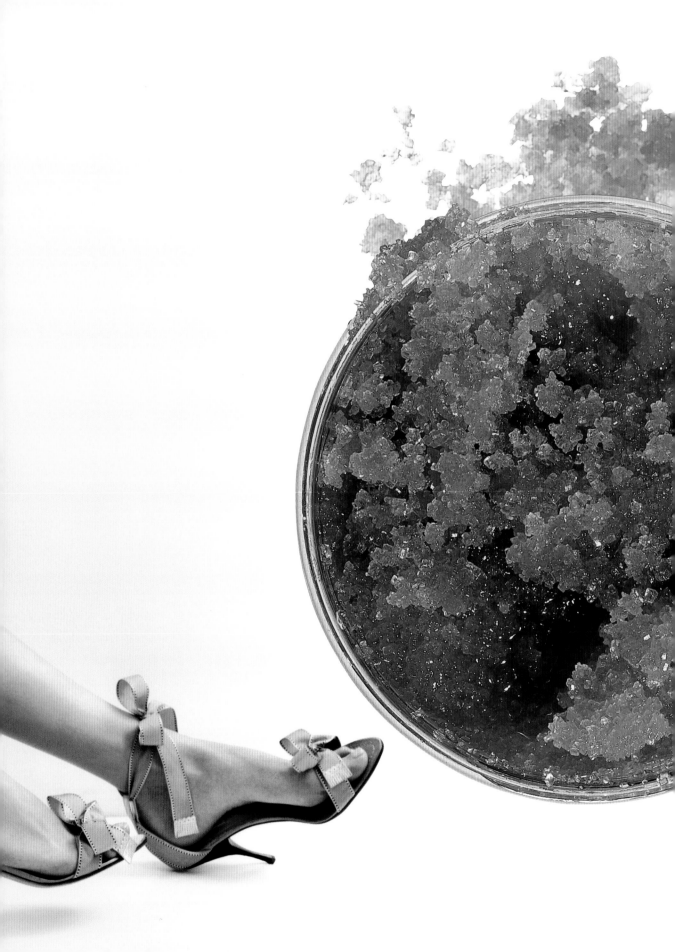

Tom Ford, the former designer for Gucci and Yves Saint Laurent, once told me that he found French women sexier than American ones. The reason was simple, he said: Americans are too clean. All those showers remove the mystery of flesh and sweat, leaving the unprovocative scent of Dial in its place.

I took no offense. As a true American, I can't go a day without washing my hair, scrubbing my skin, shaving my legs. I lather, rinse, and sometimes even repeat. A trainer at a gym nicknamed me Ivory Girl. And once in college, during a particularly long layover in an airport, I broke down and washed my hair in the sink. But for one winter when I was a student in France, I gave my loofah a rest. I lived in an ancient house that had no hot water, no shower, and no bathtub — not to mention little heat. My bedtime attire included a down jacket and three pairs of socks. By morning, a small skating rink had formed on the glass of water by my bed.

Getting clean took effort. I would either have to lean over the kitchen sink, shivering, with a washcloth and soap, or pay a few francs for admission to the municipal baths. Each bathroom there was palatial, with a massive marble tub and a robust attendant in a starched gray dress. She grunted over the polished brass faucets while I peeled off my sweater, turtleneck, and long underwear and soaked, turning on the hot water with my toe when the bath grew gray and cold. Too soon, Madame threw open the door, clapped her hands, and yanked out the drain stopper, and I would get dressed again in all those layers of wool. That bath was the most luxurious thing I'd ever experienced; its steamy comfort put me in a thick daze. But when I walked back to school, icicles formed in my hair, and I went from daily to weekly to biweekly trips.

That time in France taught me regretfully little about the *plus-que-parfait* or the works of Jean Genet. I did discover that in a pinch I could survive without washing my hair every eight hours or scouring my skin raw. And even though I briefly embraced a bit of French custom, it didn't make me feel even remotely sexy.

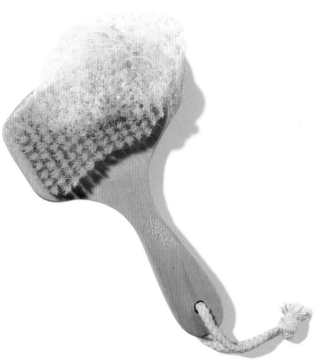

We have showering down to a science.

We used to protest when our siblings called us bossy. But considering that we're about to tell you how to take a shower, they might have had a point. Still, as simple as this morning staple seems, the right water temperature, cleansers, even the shower's duration, can really improve skin's comfort and appearance.

IN THE WINTER, it's tempting to turn an ordinary morning rinse into a half-hour steam orgy. But doing so actually breaks down the skin's lipid layer, a complex of fatty acids designed to retain moisture. You're better off turning down the heat as much as you can stand. If your teeth are chattering, at least restrict stall time to 15 minutes or less.

WE ARE BIG FANS OF BEING CLEAN, but in all likelihood, your arms and legs don't really get *that* dirty. Dermatologists say that it's only necessary to lather under your arms and you know where — the suds that slide down your body will suffice for the rest. If this sounds unsavory, consider that water does a great job of cleaning off sweat all by itself.

SOAP HAS COME A LONG WAY since that hard lump of lye used by the pioneers. Unless it's specifically labeled "deodorant" (or smells suspiciously like pine), it's probably packed with moisturizers. But if your skin is easily irritated or prone to flakiness, pass on soaps with a high amount of drying detergents like sodium laurel sulfate in favor of a creamy body wash or anything containing colloidal oatmeal — an especially soothing ingredient.

Beauty Myth

The Myth: Antiperspirant can cause cancer.

THE TRUTH: The theory that antiperspirant doesn't allow the body to sweat out toxins, which then build up in the lymph nodes, has been around for decades. (Remember Shirley MacLaine's character blaming her daughter's fatal illness on roll-on in *Terms of Endearment*?) A recent study by the Fred Hutchinson Cancer Research Center in Seattle concluded that there is no link whatsoever. Oh, and if you've heard that the aluminum in antiperspirant causes Alzheimer's, that's not true, either, according to the Alzheimer's Association. Aluminum is the third most common element on earth, after oxygen and silicon.

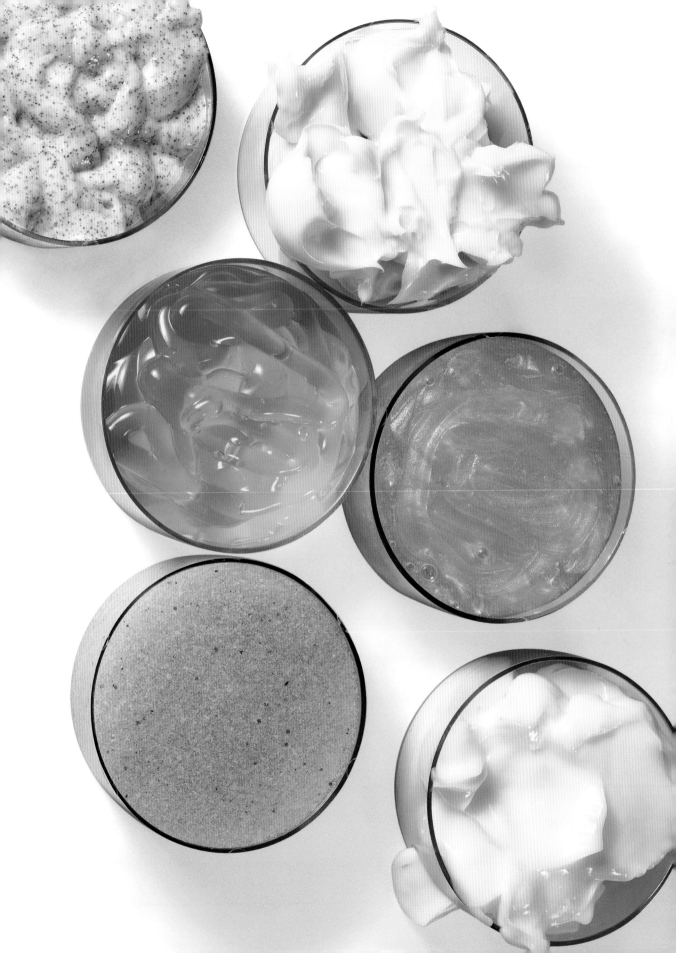

Behold the power of exfoliation.

We used to love going to the spa for a full-body scrub-down . . . until Marcia Kilgore, the founder of Bliss Spas, told us how to do it at home. It may not be as decadent as having someone buff every inch, but the results are pretty impressive.

ONCE A WEEK, before getting in the shower, dampen skin with oil by either spraying or rubbing it on. Using short, light strokes, run a firm, natural-bristle body brush over the skin, beginning at the feet and proceeding upward to make sure you don't miss anything.

STANDING IN THE SHOWER (to prevent mess), follow the same path with a thick, grainy scrub. One with sugar, salt, or tiny microbeads is better than anything with harsh shells or fruit pits. This process should feel scratchy but not painful; if you have sensitive skin, you might skip this altogether.

START A WARM — NOT HOT — SHOWER, rinse off the scrub, then apply an exfoliating body wash that contains alpha hydroxy or salicylic acid. Pay extra attention to the elbows, knees, and heels (and consider smoothing it over these parts on a daily basis). As soon as you get out of the shower, pat yourself with a towel, but leave skin slightly damp. Slather on moisturizer immediately to seal the water into your newly polished skin.

WE AREN'T HUGE FANS OF LOOFAHS or those puffy nylon scrubbers — both are serious breeding grounds for bacteria and fungi (lovely). If grainy scrubs are too hard on your skin, consider using a regular old washcloth — it's gentle, and you can just toss it into the laundry and grab a fresh one the next day.

We sometimes identify with the crocodile in that lotion commercial.

With the exception of croissants and pie crust, nothing good can come of being described as "flaky." Here's how to quench dry skin (and prevent it from becoming parched in the first place).

APPLYING MOISTURIZER OVER ROUGH SKIN is like cramming at the end of an all-night study session — nothing sinks in. Exfoliate with a grainy wash every day until skin looks less gnarly.

AS FOR THE CREAM ITSELF, dermatologists like products that deliver a one-two punch of humectants such as glycerin or hyaluronic acid (to draw water to the skin) and occlusive ingredients such as petrolatum, shea butter, or other oils (to trap water there). You can gauge how thick and rich a formula is by shaking the bottle; if you hear it sloshing around, it's too thin for truly dry skin.

Trick of the Trade

If your elbows are starting to resemble those of an elephant, try this slightly unsavory treatment (on a night when you're sleeping alone). Right before bed, cut the toes off a clean pair of cotton athletic socks, slather the elbows with Crisco, and slide the socks over the mess. The vegetable shortening is so effective at softening that it's sometimes used in hospitals to treat eczema.

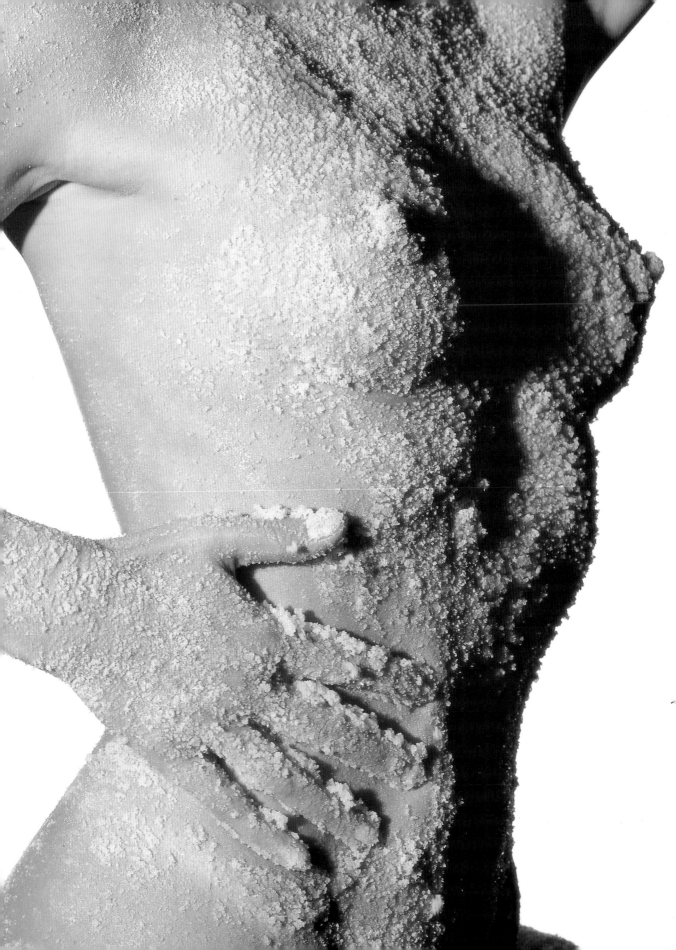

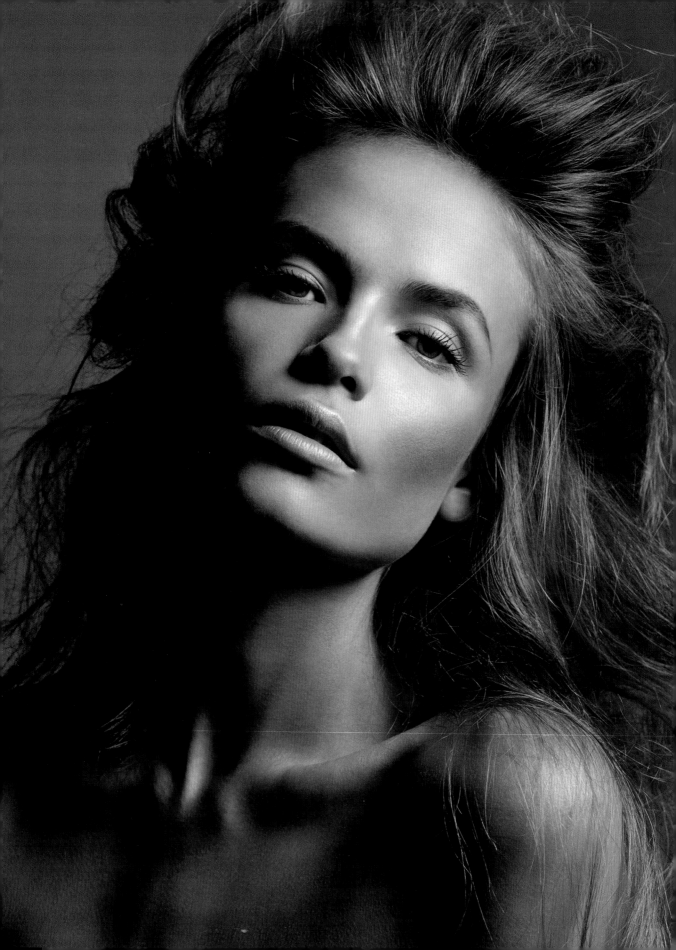

IF YOUR POOR EPIDERMIS IS SO DRY it's cracking, give those areas special attention. Dermatologists recommend slathering on a mild cortisone cream to treat itching or inflammation, followed by a heavy, petrolatum-based cream or balm twice a day. And stay far away from alpha hydroxy acids — they will burn like hellfire.

We have an advanced degree in sunscreen application.

When Malibu Barbie made her comeback after 18 years in retirement, Mattel packaged the surfer girl with her own tiny bottle of SPF 30. Judging by her bronzed skin, she's not using it correctly — like far too many of us who haphazardly slap on lotion at the beach.

AT LEAST BARBIE'S *INTENTIONS* WERE GOOD: Dermatologists say that SPF 15 doesn't cut it anymore, and recommend wearing an absolute minimum of SPF 30 when you expect to be outdoors for more than a few minutes. Just as with the face, look for a formula that offers broad-spectrum protection from both UVB (the rays that cause burning) and UVA (the ones that cause aging). Key ingredients are avobenzone (also called Parsol 1789), titanium dioxide, or zinc oxide.

FIFTEEN TO 30 MINUTES before stepping into your bikini, rub at least one ounce over the whole body, starting at the neck and working your way down. That's enough to fill a shot glass — an amount that may feel a little slimy and overwhelming at first. If you can't stand it, rub on half that amount, wait ten minutes for it to dry, and then apply a second layer. Since we've carped incessantly about wearing sunscreen on the face every day, you should already have that down. Do so now.

BEFORE YOU LEAVE THE HOUSE, check to make sure you've remembered the most often neglected areas: on the ears, behind the ears, in the crooks of the arms, between the fingers and toes, behind the knees, and on the tops of the feet.

Trick of the Trade

We once asked top dermatologists for the best advice they'd ever been given, and a surprisingly high number of them said the same thing: Apply sunscreen to the backs of your hands every day. Their paper-thin skin is one of the first places to show signs of aging.

Beauty Myth

The Myth: Waterproof sunscreen can last all day.

THE TRUTH: The term "waterproof" was banned by the FDA back in 1999 for being misleading. To be labeled "water resistant," a product must stay on for up to 40 minutes in the water or while you are sweating. Still, dermatologists say you should reapply any sunscreen every two hours, or immediately after coming out of the ocean or pool.

ONCE YOU'RE OUT THERE HAVING FUN, make sure you reapply every two hours (and every time you get out of the water, or more often if you're sweating), no matter what claims of longevity are made on the label.

We've learned that some sun damage can be reversed.

We remember our mother chasing us around the beach, dutifully reapplying sunscreen. Unfortunately, it was SPF 4. Anyone who's ever had a childhood sunburn (and possibly compounded the problem later by lying out basted in baby oil) will start to see evidence of sun damage on her chest in her early 30s. Fortunately, there are ways to fade those dark spots.

IF YOU START EARLY, up to 50 percent of damage can be gradually faded with prescription retinoids (such as Avage, Retin-A, or Renova) or TriLuma (a mix of Retin-A, skin-lightening hydroquinone, and cortisone). For sensitive skin, there's EpiQuin, a hydroquinone-and-retinol cream that slowly releases antioxidants into the skin, reducing the chance of irritation.

IF THE DAMAGE IS SEVERE ENOUGH to be described as mottled (or if money is no object), consider a dermatologic artillery. Microdermabrasion can efface spots in four to ten treatments, and the SilkPeel marries microdermabrasion with hydroquinone to work even faster. Truly stubborn brown spots (and the tiny broken blood vessels that often accompany them) can be diminished with a few blasts of a laser or a treatment called Intense Pulsed Light photorejuvenation.

We've embraced self-tanner.

We love the look of a tan but hate the possibility of living a leathery-skinned future. That's where self-tanner comes in. Here's how to get a safe, subtle glow — minus the streaks, splotches, and orange palms.

BEGIN YOUR PREPARATION with a thorough exfoliation in the shower (dry skin soaks up the color unevenly). Shaving your legs and rubbing the rest of the body with a grainy scrub, paying extra attention to rough spots like elbows and ankles, should do it. Towel-dry thoroughly, and allow skin to cool for about ten minutes. Then pull long hair up off your face into a high ponytail or bun, and dab a bit of petroleum jelly in your belly button.

IF YOU ARE USING AN AEROSOL SPRAY, spritz it directly onto the skin from about eight inches away, rubbing it in (if the label says to do so)

Beauty 911

Your self-tanner looks completely believable — except on your pumpkin-colored palms.

Since the color is only on the upper layers of skin, you can undo the damage by exfoliating. Salon pros rub their hands with salt or a halved lemon, but any scrub will do. (Nail-polish remover is also an option, but it's very drying.) For streaks on your legs or arms, scrub, rinse, wait a few minutes for skin to calm down, then reapply tanning cream only on the exfoliated area. If you use a pea-size amount and make sure you've blended it in, you should be all set.

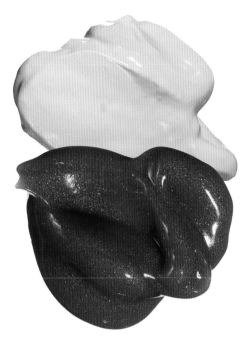

after finishing each body part. Otherwise, apply a quarter-size blob of self-tanning lotion at a time. Massage it in with horizontal swoops, then vertical, proceeding slowly from the bottoms of your legs to your neck and making sure not to forget commonly overlooked areas like the neck or under your breasts and butt. Save the following body parts for last: the tops of the feet and hands; the insides of the arms; and the armpits, heels, ankles, toes, knees, and elbows. A swipe with what's left over on your palms should suffice for those areas.

WASH YOUR PALMS AND FINGERS, and scrub your nails immediately with soap and water, then blot excess cream from the knees and elbows with a tissue. Wait at least 20 minutes for the self-tanner to dry before getting dressed, holding your head high as long as you can bear, to avoid dark spots in the creases of the neck. Put on an old, loose T-shirt and dark underwear, and go to bed. The next morning, don't rub your skin too hard with a towel after showering; apply moisturizer twice a day until your next application (roughly three days later).

Cheater's Guide

When we can't be bothered to self-tan but still don't want to look both pale *and* dull, we reach for our secret weapon: body shimmer. It doesn't have to be as Vegas as it sounds, honest: Just take a shimmer lotion (one that's silvery for pale skin or golden for olive or dark complexions), and cut it with a little regular moisturizer first. Rub it onto areas where light would usually hit, like the shoulders, collarbones, forearms, and shins. And don't forget to add a little swipe of glimmery powder to the eyelids or cheekbones — a shiny body with a totally matte face is spooky.

Damage Control

If you've stupidly let yourself sizzle in the sun, all you can do is try to minimize the consequences. Start by cooling off the skin: After a burn, blood rushes to the surface, so applying a cold compress or taking a cool bath for ten minutes will help constrict blood vessels. After that, skip topical anesthetics like Solarcaine (which numb rather than treat inflammation), and pop two aspirin instead — it actually prevents further redness as well as relieves pain. Once puffiness has subsided, apply a vitamin E– or C–based cream twice a day to keep the area hydrated. It will probably still peel, but keep your hands off — the dead layer protects the damaged skin below.

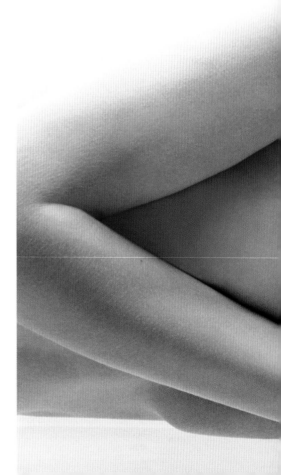

We hate being reminded we've out-grown our birthday suits.

While we may wish for a magic cream that will make them disappear, stretch marks are among the most intractable skin problems. You can attempt to minimize them, but don't expect a miracle.

THE BEST WAY TO COMBAT STRETCH MARKS is to catch them early. Application of topical prescription-strength retinoids, such as Retin-A, Renova, or Avage, when the marks are still red may shrink them in size. (Cocoa butter and vitamin E won't do a thing.) For the time being, there is no cream that helps the older white marks, so you might as well wish for world peace when you're leaning over that birthday cake.

LASER TREATMENTS MAY HAVE A BIGGER IMPACT on your credit card balance than on stretch marks. Pulsed dye lasers, like the Vbeam and VStar, zap redness in young marks; infrared lasers, like the Smoothbeam, build collagen to refine the texture of white ones. But an honest dermatologist will tell you that a 20 percent improvement, after three to five sessions at up to $500 apiece, is about the best you'll get. The excimer and BClear lasers seem to hold the most promise; they've been proven to repigment white marks — though it takes 10 to 18 sessions, plus maintenance zaps in the future.

If there were a cure for cellulite, our thighs would be smooth (damn it).

More than 70 percent of women have cellulite, according to the last study we saw. We'd like to smack the 30 percent who don't.

THAT ORANGE-PEEL TEXTURE is the dimpling of fatty tissue under the skin. Doctors don't know exactly what causes it, but think it's some mix of metabolic, circulatory, and genetic factors. In other words, the concept of flushing the body of impurities may sell spa appointments, but it doesn't affect cellulite, which has absolutely nothing to do with toxins or blocked lymphatic flow.

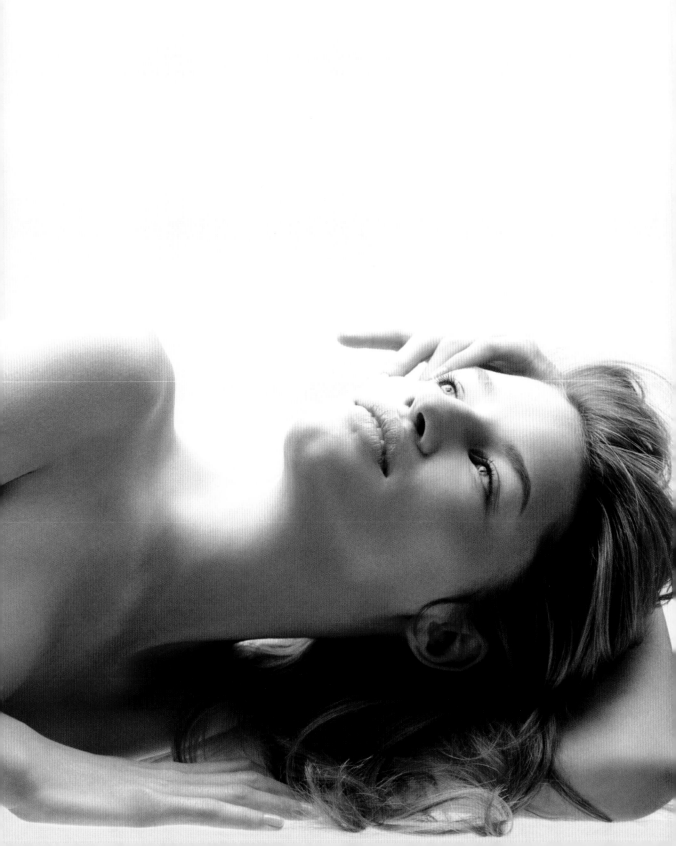

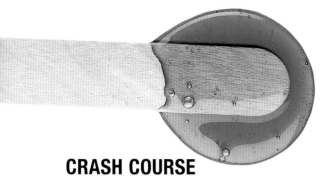

CRASH COURSE
How to Do a Home Bikini Wax

The first time you wax at home, you're all but guaranteed to get wax everywhere and curse loudly. Here's how to minimize the mess (and the pain) while you save a little money.

GET READY . . . Most home waxing kits are tricky. Avoid cold waxes altogether, since they barely work and are impossibly sticky. Better to hit the beauty-supply store for a professional wax warmer (it's about $50), honey-based wax, cloth strips, and tongue depressors. Take two ibuprofen an hour ahead of time, cover the floor with newspaper (since wax will inevitably spill), and then strip off your underwear (wax isn't easy to wash out).

GET SET . . . Sit on a stool or the edge of the bathtub, scooting your butt as far forward as possible, and spread your legs. Use nail scissors to trim hair to a quarter inch, then dust powder all over the area to keep wax from bonding to the skin. Be sure to test the wax temperature on your wrist before you proceed — it should be warm, not scalding.

GO. Dip a tongue depressor into the wax, and spread a thin layer on a one-by-two-inch section of hair, following the growth. Press on a cloth strip, pull skin taut, and take a big breath as you pull off the strip. Working in small sections will allow you to see what you're doing and (along with that ibuprofen) make it a bit less painful.

SOOTHE THE SKIN. Dab baby oil on any spots where wax got stuck. Then soak a cotton ball in warm chamomile tea, and hold it on the skin to calm the area. Rub on an aloe-based gel or hydrocortisone cream, and congratulate yourself — you did it, and it will only get easier.

CELLULITE CREAMS HAVE LONG CONTAINED ingredients like caffeine and seaweed, which reduce water in the skin and make the area look firmer. To the bikini-wearing public, this means a slight tightening that only lasts while the cream is on the skin. (You weren't planning on actually swimming in that suit, were you?) Even the latest ingredients can't turn skin from lumpy to lithe, but they are better at hiding it. Retinoids, the only group of ingredients proven to build collagen, even out the skin so that fat bulges are harder to see. DMAE is a natural anti-inflammatory derived from fish that seems to have promise in firming skin over time. And forskolin, derived from a root long used in Ayurvedic medicine, has recently caused a stir in the laboratory by triggering lipolysis, a process that causes fat cells to shrink. But while plenty of women rave about these creams, we've yet to see any significant improvement after using them.

IN-OFFICE PROCEDURES for cellulite abound, and keeping track of them and their claims is practi-

Trick of the Trade

To minimize scarring from a new cut or scrape, don't reach for a vitamin E capsule. A recent study showed that vitamin E oil was no better at healing than moisturizers and that it even caused irritation on some people. Instead, dermatologists insist on keeping the wound moist (your body will supply the fluid), applying a topical antibiotic ointment every day to prevent infection, and covering it with a watertight bandage until the wound closes. Then switch to the scar-reducing tension pads sold at the drugstore. They work by applying microscopic pressure, which counteracts the body's tendency to produce more scar tissue. And keep in mind that UV exposure makes a scar infinitely worse — cover up until you can apply sunscreen.

cally a full-time job. Some doctors are intrigued by the FDA-approved TriActive device, which combines suction massage and diode lasers to smooth the puckering of cellulite by shrinking fat cells and loosening deep fibrous tissue. For short-term results (think two or three days), there is the wacky-sounding Ionithermie procedure, in which the skin is coated with clay to help conduct electricity to dimpled areas.

MOST EXPERTS RECOMMEND a decidedly more low-tech approach: self-tanner. They all agree that cellulite looks worse when you're pale and pasty.

Body acne isn't just for teenagers.

Many women suffer from the old "if you can't see it, it doesn't exist" delusion about acne on the back. When you're ready to accept that zits pop up in places other than your face, here's what to do:

FOR MILD TO MODERATE CASES, dermatologists suggest washing with a salicylic acid cleanser, especially after working out or applying hair conditioner, to unclog pores, get rid of pimples, and prevent new ones. (Those with more persistent zits may want to ask their doctor for a prescription acne wash with benzoyl peroxide or sulfur.) Then apply a topical benzoyl peroxide cream to blemishes before bed.

WHEN ACNE IS MORE SEVERE, doctors are increasingly reaching for lasers, which can wipe out stubborn breakouts in as little as two to three visits (unfortunately, it's expensive). The Smoothbeam laser can treat deep acne and old scars; the Vbeam eases redness; and photodynamic therapy is best for large areas.

Shaving 101

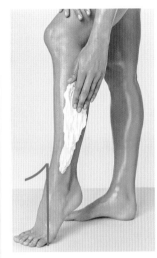

LATHER
Allow at least three minutes in the shower for warm water to penetrate and soften the hair follicle before spreading a layer of shaving cream or gel over the entire leg — lathering against the direction of the hair growth. For sensitive skin, try a formula with soothing vitamin E, aloe, or allantoin. Glycerin and panthenol will moisturize dry skin, and those prone to ingrowns can benefit from a benzoyl peroxide or salicylic acid formula.

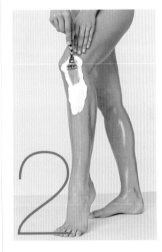

SHAVE
Prop up one leg with your knee bent so you can reach your ankle. Glide a sharp, multiblade razor over the skin, starting just above the ankle and working upward in six- to eight-inch sections. Rinse the razor between each stroke. To shave the knees and ankles, put both feet on the ground, and bend at the waist, gently pulling the skin taut. (Replace the blade after three shaves.)

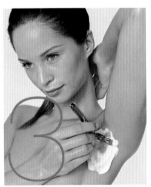

FINE TUNE
Because underarm hairs grow in multiple directions, you have to shave at different angles. Raise the arm, apply shaving cream, and move the blade upward, then downward, then across, rinsing it clean and relathering with shaving cream after every few strokes.

FIVE TOP TIPS:

Fragrance

Women tread a fine line when applying a scent: Spritz on too little, and you might as well be wearing nothing; pour on too much, and you may find co-workers gasping for air. Here's how to choose a scent that suits you, and how to wear it well:

1 It's easy to reach sensory overload in the perfume aisle at a department store. Consider rounding up a batch of scent strips (or better yet, samples) and trying them at home before you buy. When sniffing, clear your head by sticking your nose in your sleeve or in a bag of coffee between strips (many stores now offer the beans).

2 Once you've identified a contender, dab just a bit on one or two places, like a wrist and the inside of the opposite elbow. It takes about ten minutes for the scent to mix with your skin chemistry, but also wait to see how it mellows or changes through the day. It's OK if it smells different at sun-down — as long as you like the results.

3 To keep fragrance from simply wafting away, the pros recommend layering it on — for example, use the body wash in the shower paired with a few dabs of eau de parfum (a con-centrated formula), or rub on the body lotion followed by the eau de toilette (a lighter spray). Just note that two layers is plenty; three is overkill. In general, anyone within arm's reach should be able to catch a subtle hint of your scent.

4 If you've spritzed yourself one (or ten) times too many, you don't have to jump in the shower. Alcohol or witch hazel dabbed on the wrist or any other bombed-out body part will remove even oil-based formulas.

5 To keep from overdosing, switch fragrances from time to time — your nose can become desensitized to your sig-nature scent, and when you suddenly have to put on twice as much to be able to smell it yourself, you risk overpower-ing others.

Beauty Myth

The Myth: Rubbing your wrists together destroys molecules in your perfume and changes the scent.

THE TRUTH: OK, we have to cop to having written this in the magazine ourselves. More than once. Finally an astute reader with a doctorate in chemistry wrote in and pointed out that if it were that easy to crush single molecules, her job would be a lot easier. Good point, Margie Topp from the Netherlands. From now on we'll rub to our heart's content.

Trick of the Trade

As pretty as those little bottles look on the shelf, protect your perfume portfolio by keeping it out of the bathroom. The heat and humidity from daily show-ers can make certain scents go bad, and alter the notes of others. Most perfumers store theirs in the refrigerator.

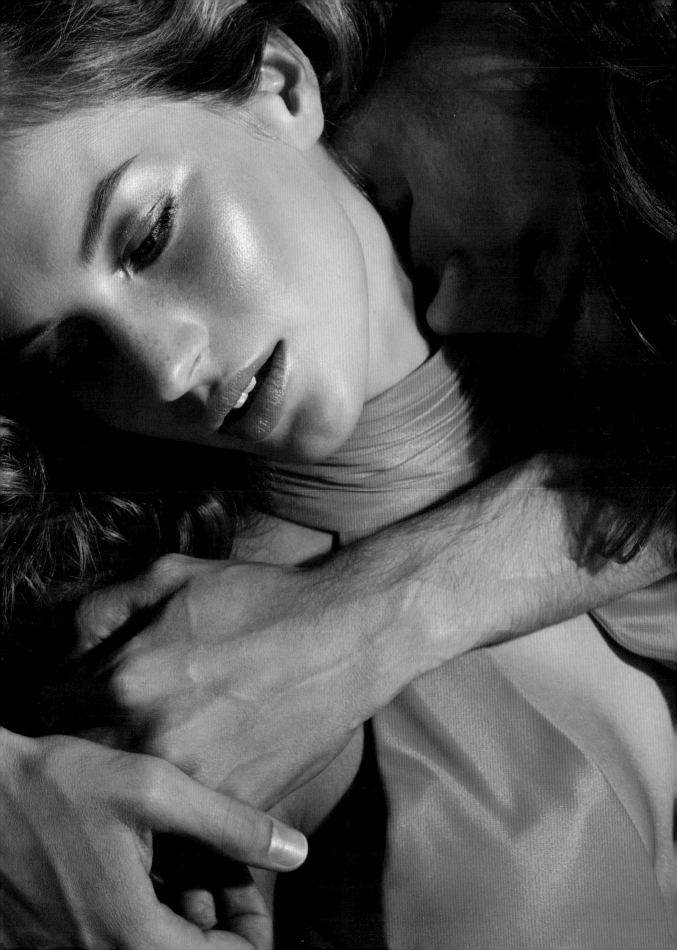

The 10 Commandments

Keep showers as cool as possible
to prevent moisture loss.

Banish flakes by exfoliating at
least once a week.

Choose a washcloth over
loofahs and puffs (which
are breeding grounds for
bacteria and fungi).

Pay special attention to
rough spots — they won't
smooth out without
daily scrubs.

Apply lotion or cream
immediately after bathing,
while skin is still damp.

Layer on fragrance if you
want it to last.

Protect against sun damage
by applying the equivalent of
a shot glass of sunscreen.

Silvery stretch marks are impossible to get rid of, but you can minimize newer pink ones with laser
treatments.

Don't bother with cellulite
creams unless you're OK with
small, fleeting results.

Self-tanner can mask a multitude
of skin problems, including veins,
age spots, even cellulite.

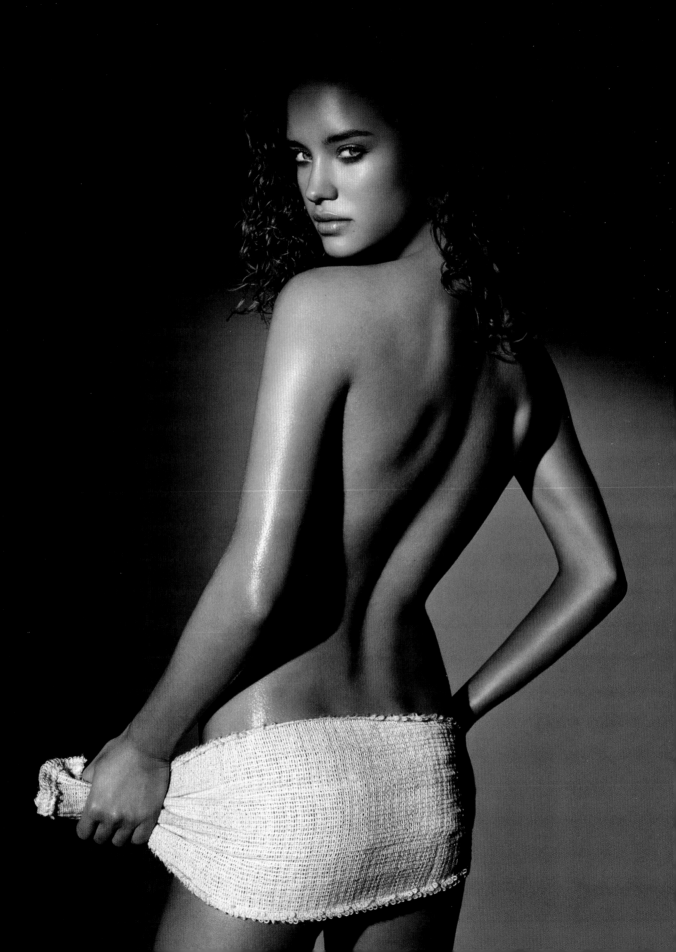

Acknowledgments

This book is a result of the energy and hard work of *Allure*'s editors, writers, designers, and assistants. My deepest thanks go especially to Sarah Van Boven, Kristin Perrotta, Paul Cavaco, Nadine McCarthy, Andrew Wilkes, Marie Jones, and David DeNicolo.

I am enormously grateful to the photographers for their generosity and vision: Richard Burbridge, Roger Cabello, Regan Cameron, Walter Chin, Patrick Demarchelier, Greg Kadel, Rennio Maifredi, Wayne Maser, Nicolas Moore, Carter Smith, Bill Steele, David Stesner, Mario Testino, Michael Thompson, and Franz Walderdorff.

I thank the makeup artists and hairstylists who are *Allure*'s rocket scientists: Scott Andrew, the late Kevyn Aucoin, Bobbi Brown, Linda Cantello, Chrisanne Davis, Sharon Dorram-Krause, Frédéric Fekkai, Garren, Odile Gilbert, Sally Hershberger, Brad Johns, Harry Josh, Louis Licari, River Lloyd, Kevin Mancuso, Stephane Marais, Pat McGrath, Chris McMillan, Laura Mercier, François Nars, Serge Normant, Oribe, Dick Page, Renée Patronik, Jimmy Paul, Guido Palau, Tom Pecheux, Orlando Pita, Eugene Souleiman, and Gucci Westman.

My team and I hound and dog and generally chew up the valuable time of the country's top dermatologists and cosmetics chemists, and they never complain. My thanks go to Lisa Donofrio, who vetted this book, Leslie Baumann, Fredric Brandt, Doris J. Day, Jeffrey Dover, Howard Fein, Kathy Fields, Jeannette Graf, Dennis Gross, Karyn Grossman, Jim Hammer, Yash Kamath, Mary P. Lupo, Nick Morante, Darrell Rigel, Katie Rodan, Ava T. Shamban, James Spencer, Mort Westman, and Patricia Wexler.

Thank you to Mandy Aftel, Chandler Burr, Frédéric Malle, Jo Malone, and Harry Slatkin. To Maribeth Madron, Eliza Petrescu, and Anastasia Soare. To Cindy Barshop, Marcia Kilgore, Nance Mitchell, and Lidia Tivichi. To Ji Baek, Sheril Bailey, Jin Soon Choi, Elisa Ferri, Deborah Lippmann, and Bernadette Thompson. To the models who put the beauty in the beauty book: Leilani Bishop, Gisele Bündchen, Michelle Buswell, Naomi Campbell, Carmen Maria Hillestad, Liya Kebede, Missy Rayder, Caroline Ribeiro, Julia Stegnor, Amber Valletta, Linda Vojtova, Marija Vujovic, Anne Vyalitsyne, and Jacquetta Wheeler.

To my bosses, past and present: Karen Anderegg, the late Carrie Donovan, the late Alexander Liberman, S. I. Newhouse, Jr., James Truman, and Tom Wallace.

Thank you to Jill Cohen, Doug Turshen, Betty Wong, and Karyn Gerhard at Bulfinch.

To my incredibly good-humored and graceful assistant, Liana Marraro, and former assistant, Patricia Tortolani.

And most of all, thank you, Charlie, Charlie, and Webster.

Photo Credits

COVER: Franz Walderdorff.

TITLE PAGE, page 3: Roger Cabello.

CONTENTS, page 5: Michael Thompson.

INTRODUCTION, page 7: Franz Walderdorff. Page 8, from left: Courtesy of subject (3), Keith King. Page 9, from left: Cutty McGill, Denis Reggie, Patrick McMullan.

CHAPTER 1, SKIN CARE, page 10: Roger Cabello. Page 11: Patric Shaw. Page 15: Nicolas Moore. Page 16: Greg Kadel. Page 17: Roe Ethridge (3). Page 18: Roger Cabello. Page 20: Roger Cabello. Page 21: Carter Smith. Page 22: Andrew McKim. Page 27: Michael Thompson.

CHAPTER 2, SKIN PROBLEMS, page 28: Michael Thompson. Page 29: Roger Cabello. Page 33: David Stesner. Page 34: David Cook. Page 41: Nicolas Moore.

CHAPTER 3, FACE, page 42: Roger Cabello. Page 43: Regan Cameron. Page 46: Roger Cabello. Page 47: Rennio Maifredi. Page 48: David Stesner, Roger Cabello (stills). Page 50: Michael Thompson. Page 51: Roger Cabello. Page 52: Roger Cabello. Page 53: Michael Thompson. Page 54, from left: David Cook, Roger Cabello. Page 56: Roger Cabello. Page 57: Carter Smith. Page 58: Roger Cabello. Page 61: Roger Cabello. Page 63: Michael Thompson. Page 65: Michael Thompson.

CHAPTER 4, EYES, page 66: David Cook. Page 67: Carter Smith. Page 70: Roger Cabello. Page 71: Nicolas Moore. Page 72: Roger Cabello (stills). Page 73: David Stesner (3). Page 75: Franz Walderdorff. Page 77: David Cook. Page 78: Patrick Demarchelier. Page 81: Mario Testino. Page 83: Regan Cameron.

CHAPTER 5, LIPS, page 84: Roger Cabello. Page 85: Walter Chin. Page 88: Roger Cabello. Page 89: Carter Smith. Page 90: Roger Cabello. Page 94: Wayne Maser. Page 95: David Stesner. Page 97: Michael Thompson.

CHAPTER 6, NAILS, page 98: Wayne Maser. Page 99: Roger Cabello. Page 102: Bill Steele. Page 103: Patric Shaw. Page 104: Wayne Maser. Page 106: Roger Cabello. Page 107: David Stesner (3). Page 108: Roger Cabello. Page 111: Richard Burbridge. Page 112: Roger Cabello. Page 113: Regan Cameron. Page 115: Richard Burbridge.

CHAPTER 7, HAIRCUT AND COLOR, page 116: Roger Cabello. Page 117: Regan Cameron. Page 120: Nicolas Moore. Page 121: Michael Thompson. Page 124: Michael Thompson, Roger Cabello (stills). Page 125: Walter Chin. Page 127: Rennio Maifredi. Page 128: Michael Thompson. Page 130: Regan Cameron. Page 131: David Stesner (3). Page 133: Patrick Demarchelier.

CHAPTER 8, HAIR CARE AND STYLE, page 134: Carter Smith. Page 135: Roger Cabello. Page 139: Patrick Demarchelier. Page 141: David Stesner (3). Page 142: Patrick Demarchelier. Page 146: Roger Cabello (stills). Page 147: Bill Diodato (stills). Page 149: Carter Smith. Page 150: Michael Thompson. Page 151: Aimee Levy (illustration). Page 153: Carter Smith.

CHAPTER 9, SALONS AND SPAS, page 154: Wayne Maser. Page 159: David Stesner. Page 160: Greg Kadel. Page 164: Tesh. Page 167: Wayne Maser.

CHAPTER 10, BODY, page 168: Mario Testino. Page 169: Roger Cabello. Page 172: Roger Cabello. Page 173: Roger Cabello. Page 175: Michael Thompson. Page 176: Michael Thompson. Page 179: Roger Cabello. Page 181: Michael Thompson. Page 182: Roger Cabello. Page 183: David Stesner (3). Page 185: Michael Thompson. Page 187: Wayne Maser.

Index

BULFINCH PRESS

Hachette Book Group USA
1271 Avenue of the Americas
New York, NY 10020

Visit our Web site at
www.bulfinchpress.com

First Edition: October 2006

ISBN-10: 0-8212-5779-X
ISBN-13: 978-0-8212-5779-1
LCCN: 2006924151

Design by Doug Turshen with David Huang

PRINTED IN SINGAPORE